Healing America

Books by Roger J. Bulger, MD

In Search of the Modern Hippocrates

Technology, Bureaucracy, and Healing in America

The Quest for Mercy –
The Forgotten Ingredient in Health Care Reform

The Honorable Paul G. Rogers –
A Portrait in Leadership and a Fighter for Health

Physician Philosopher – The Philosophical Foundation of Medicine
Essays by Dr. Edmund Pellegrino
(as co-editor)

Healing America

Hope, Mercy, Justice and Autonomy in the American Health Care System

Roger J. Bulger, MD

PROSPECTA PRESS

Published by
Prospecta Press
P.O. Box 3131
Westport, CT 06880
(203) 454-4454
www.prospectapress.com

Paperback ISBN: 978-1-935212-21-8
E-book ISBN: 978-1-935212-20-1

Book and cover design by Barbara Aronica-Buck

Printed in the United States of America

First Printing: July 2010

10 9 8 7 6 5 4 3 2 1

Dedication

To Doris and Roy Brunjes, friends of mine for over sixty years and at whose wedding in 1955 I served as best man. With their welcoming natures, optimism, integrity, and upbeat endurance they have lived exemplary lives both professionally and socially—even in the face, later in life, of serious chronic disease and significant disability. For myself and the many others lucky enough to know them, I thank them for being such wonderful models of how to live happily.

To all those who, whether they know it or not, have enabled this effort throughout the years—intellectually, substantively, and otherwise—including especially the following: John J. McGovern, MD; June Osborn, MD; Edmund Pellegrino, MD; the Honorable Paul G. Rogers, John R. Hogness, MD; William G. Anlyan, MD; Donald S. Fredrickson, MD; Leigh Cluff, MD; Linda Clever, MD; the Honorable Louis Sullivan, MD; the Honorable John Edward Porter, Julius Richmond, MD; Admiral David Satcher, MD; Ruth Bulger, PhD; Harvey Estes, MD; Eugene Stead, MD; Lawrence Green, PhD; Guido Majno, MD; David Mechanic, PhD; Stanley Reiser, MD; Robert G. Petersdorf, MD; Arnold S. Relman, MD; Uwe Rhinehart, PhD; Leon Eisenberg, MD; Henry Foster, MD; John Stoeckle, MD;

Jane Henney, MD; Linda Aiken, PhD, RN; Elaine Larson, PhD, RN; Kay Andreoli, DSN, RN; John McDermott, PhD; John Ruffin, PhD; John Sherris, MD; Patricia Starck, PhD, RN; Lawrence Tancredi, MD; John Benson, MD; Virginia Tilden, PhD, RN; Ronald B. Miller, MD; B. Harvey Minchew, MD; and Donald Wilson, MD.

Contents

PART II
Elements for Successful Adaptation
in the Twenty-first Century

Foreword

The initial stimulus for this book was a question fifteen years ago asking the author what college students should know about medical careers. Unwilling to rest with what he considered a partial answer to this inquiry, Roger Bulger has delivered a complete and informative look at not only the organizational, scientific, academic, and technical aspects of the practice of medicine, but also the emotional and personal characteristics needed in physicians and other health professionals. Additionally, he addresses the major problematic issues facing health care in the United States, doing so with a depth of understanding that will be valuable to both health professionals and patients alike. He gives readers a broad sociological perspective of health care that reaches back to the Hippocratic oath and concludes with a provocative system to evaluate the performance of individuals, teams, and organizations in the modern health care system.

The product of considerable research, thoroughness, and erudition, the book fulfills the author's intent, set forth in the introduction, to provide the reader with "a basic guide to the issues affecting health care in our society."

Having spent some forty years as a physician in clinical settings, I was struck with Dr. Bulger's attention to the need for certain personal characteristics in a medical practitioner. He notes that mutual trust forms the foundation of the doctor-patient relationship and is essential for this relationship to be fully professional and ethical. Likewise, honesty is critical for the ongoing relationship to grow and function properly. Dr. Bulger also stresses the importance of health professionals' commitment to personal service and community service as well as a high level of competence. He has provided an oath of the modern Hippocrates, which includes the need to "promise my patients competence, integrity, candor, personal commitment to their best interests, compassion, and absolute discretion and confidentiality within the law."

Realizing the relatively stressful life of the clinician, Dr. Bulger discusses the necessity for periodic personal assessments of one's physical energy levels, emotional reserves, and the adequacy of each for meeting one's responsibilities. This assessment obviously involves an awareness of one's personal sources of energy and how to replenish them. Dr. Bulger notes that service to others can often be a significant source of satisfaction and energy. An active professional curiosity, in my experience, can also be such a source.

The aspects of personal character discussed in this book need to be manifest through honest insights and self-awareness. Dr. Bulger's astute commentary brings to mind lines from Shakespeare that apply well to today's health professionals and the problematical situations they regularly encounter:

> This above all, to thine own self be true,
> And it must follow as the night the day,
> Thou cans't not then be false to any man.
> *Hamlet*, act I, scene iii

Most important in relation to potential changes in the health care system, Dr. Bulger reminds us of the need for yet another human characteristic: "It would be a tragedy, just when we have so many effective scientific therapies at hand, for policy makers to negotiate away the element of compassion, leaving this critical dimension of healing solely to unscientific healers or to no one."

Keep reading. You are in for a most informative and enjoyable book.

B. H. Minchew, MD

Introduction

When Doctors Become Patients

I daydream a lot—always have! The other day, for example, I dreamed that I was the   chairman of the board of my own personal health care company.

I had a lot of power as board chair, overseeing the medical and business professionals responsible for my health care. I dreamed that I was able to make my computer work, and when I pressed "1*" my personal health care company's website popped onto the screen with the American flag flying in the background. From the home page I clicked on to a list of my company's primary staff and essential team members. My primary care clinician served as chief executive officer (CEO) except when I placed that function in the hands of one of several specialists, including dentists, psychologists, advanced-practice nurses, physician assistants, pharmacists, and physical and occupational therapists. At the click of the mouse, I could email any, some, or all of them with questions or requests for appointments. At my discretion, they could have access to my record and could communicate with one another about my health care. In the event that I could not make decisions, my designated health care proxy would serve as interim board chair.

My fantasy continued to the next website pages, which covered business, financial, and health information. The business and financial information pages allowed me to guesstimate the total projected cost and personal out-of-pocket charges for any treatment or hospitalization. I could also make similar financial forecasts for one year of care for any specific chronic disease.

The health information page gave me access to authoritative studies of the effectiveness of various treatments and diagnostic options. From this page, I could query my health care team and designated specialists for comment. Just as I was being called back to reality, I glimpsed a tantalizing title for the concluding section of my personal health information and business record: "A Human Values Model for Evaluation of Personal Health Care Companies."

In brief, this book attempts to explore, describe, and complete the background for that daydream. The book concerns the care of patients and the care of society as a whole. It is about the healing relationship that can occur between patients and health care professionals; and between patients, groups of potential patients, and the institutions and organizations charged with providing health care, public health, and health promotion services. It has the audacity to look at what is good about our current health care enterprise in an era of specialization, when single physicians no longer provide most or all the necessary services for their patients. It paints an optimistic picture of what our twenty-first-century health care can become in the years ahead, when America finds the will and the way to provide good health care for all its citizens.

Many experts in medicine, health, economics, and societal affairs have addressed the complex health care challenges that confront us in this era of rapid change and uncertain futures. I enter this discussion because my most recent experience as a physician-patient has convinced me that the paternalistic doctor-patient relationship of fifty years ago has morphed—through the concepts of shared decision making and collaborative care—to make my daydream the emerging model of the future. That model resembles a small corporation dedicated to caring for the health of one individual. If the chair of the board of this corporation is the patient, then the CEOs and executives are physicians, dentists, nurses, or other providers of care at various times. The concept of the patient as board chair means that the board overseeing an individual's health care enterprise, so to speak, must include more than medical professionals. It must expand—and medical professionals and administrators must facilitate its expansion—to include patients, their families, and others designated by patients or those responsible for their care. I have written this book for all these potential board members, in the hope of providing a basic guide to the issues affecting health care in our society.

In addition to having been both a clinician and a patient, I have been a medical-school teacher and administrator who thought at first that teaching medical students covered the necessary bases to secure the future of medical care. Over time, I recognized that the health care team extends beyond doctors to include nurses, dentists, public health and allied health professionals, and health care administrators. Furthermore, educating the members of these groups only within their individual professions will not meet the long-term challenge of providing the various services our citizens need.

Health care is a means, not an end, and this book is ultimately about creating a healthier society—without the gross injustice inherent in tens of millions of Americans being uninsured or significantly underinsured—by improving the relationships among patients, medical professionals, and health care institutions and agencies. These relationships are all evolving rapidly under the pressure of many forces, not least the fact that health care represents almost one-fifth of our national economy. Advances in biological research and technological innovation present us with unparalleled challenges in workforce organizational development. I write this book as a participant observer of these ongoing changes over the past half-century—as a physician, teacher, researcher, administrator, and, most important, a patient who has survived three life-threatening illnesses, thanks to the care and compassionate concern of medical professionals, family, and friends.

I have lived and worked all over the country in a fortunate variety of roles during the five decades I have spent in the health care arena. From 1960 to 1972, I was a clinician concerned with individual patients and a professor of medicine and community health sciences, first at the University of Washington in Seattle and then at Duke University in Durham, North Carolina. From 1967 to 1970, I was also medical director of the University of Washington Hospital, and from 1970 to 1972, associate director of the Durham, North Carolina, Veterans Administration Hospital; associate dean at Duke Medical School; and dean of the Duke University School for the Allied Health Sciences. From 1972 to 1976, I served as the first executive officer of the Institute of Medicine of the National Academy of Sciences. From 1976 to 1978, I was chancellor of the University of Massachusetts Medical Center at Worcester, Massachusetts, and dean of its medical school. From 1978 to 1988, I was president of the University of Texas Health Science Center at Houston. From 1988 to 2005, I was president and chief executive officer of the Association of Academic Health Centers, the organization that brings all the academic health center leaders in the country together. From 2005 to 2007, I came out of retirement to work with Dr. John Ruffin, the director of the National Center for Minority Health and Health Disparities at the National Institutes of Health, first as a consultant and then as interim deputy director.

In all my administrative jobs, I strove to explore and write about at least one major issue each year that arose from my experiences as an administrator. I hoped in part to demonstrate that adopting an administrative role need not become a denial of, or separation from, intellectual life. I thus wrote about the forces impinging on the health professions and their educational and clinical organizations. I am not a brilliant polymath, however. Rather, I am a plodding generalist investigator who has kept trying to understand our strengths and weaknesses as health professionals and how to improve the health of our patients, our nation, and ultimately populations around the world, particularly in developing countries.

The major illnesses I have experienced in my own life have dramatically influenced my view of American health care and the societal obligations of health professionals. These experiences and those of several other physician-patients underlie much of what this book has to say.

I begin with the issues, challenges, and values of the physician in a healing relationship with another human being we refer to as the "patient." Later, I argue for the adoption of these same values as the basis for the multimembered health care team. I go so far as to propose the concept of a "healing institution" or "healing organization," including a set of benchmarks for assessing such an entity. The last chapter describes a vision for the twenty-first-century American health care system, which from my point of view is neither utopian nor impossible but well within our reach. This vision expresses my belief that making patients the leaders of their health care teams, the board chairs of their own virtual health care companies, should be the centerpiece of our revolutionized and universally available health care system.

Some determined, knowledgeable, well-insured patients are already transforming their health care in this way, along with forward-thinking medical professionals. The essential pieces for continuing the process are in place or developing rapidly. What hangs in the balance is whether we can find the will to extend this capability throughout the health care system, for the benefit of patients, medical professionals, and our society as a whole.

Part I

The Core
of Health Care

Chapter 1

A Physician's Lessons from Being a Patient

In the winter of 1954–55, as a college senior looking forward to entering medical school, I asked a middle-aged physician named Donald S. Gates what was special to him in his practice of internal medicine. He said, "Some of the most moving and significant moments are when I am with patients who are consciously confronting the reality of their own imminent death."

Dr. Gates's words anchored themselves in my memory and emerged repeatedly when I was with patients facing life's end. Yet I never thought of his words in terms of my own mortality until the summer of 2007, when I became the patient facing—and expecting—imminent death. This was so even though I had faced the same prospect from the same disease, mixed-cell lymphoma, in 1994. My two bouts with cancer were not my first brush with a life-threatening illness, however.

A Child's View of Illness

One afternoon in 1940, when I was seven years old, I came home from school at the usual time with a sore throat and fever. In an hour or so my throat seemed to be closing up and I emitted a harsh, high-pitched wheeze with every breath. By this time my mother had come home from her fifth-grade public school teaching job, and she immediately called Dr. Cirillo, a general practitioner-surgeon who had his office nearby. During the several minutes we waited for him, I saw the look on the face of my six-years-older brother, Bill, grow anguished with fear, near horror, and concern, as my breathing became more and more labored.

Dr. Cirillo took me directly to the hospital, where he got me through the immediate problem by doing a tracheotomy that allowed me to breathe. My technical diagnosis, as I now know, was acute streptococcal epiglossitis with severe laryngeal stridor. The strep throat was still raging when double pneumonia also hit.

Over the next days in the hospital in Queens, New York, where we lived, I heard several people say I would die. I had the last rites of the Roman Catholic Church, a sacrament I knew about, having prepared for and received my first communion just before getting sick.

Although these experiences convinced me that I was going to die, I do not recall feeling great distress or suffering very much in any way during this episode. I had no doubt of my parents' and my brother's positive feelings for me before this, but I was now catapulted from being the youngest and most junior in the family constellation to the center of the emotional stage. I received enormous attention and loving concern from them all.

Three vivid images from that illness remain with me. The first is my father lying on a pallet about twelve inches higher than the one I lay on, as we were connected vein to vein so that blood could flow from him to me. No one explained what was happening or why, but I knew my father was directly involved in trying to save my life.

Second is the vision of my pediatrician, Dr. Shapiro, sitting observing me for long periods, head in hand, during the few days of the recover-or-not crisis in the course of the bacterial pneumonia in both my lungs. At the time, it seemed to my family and me that his mere presence helped. Years later, the sight of him at my bedside came instantly to mind when I saw an illustration in a medical book of Luke Fildes's iconic painting, *The Doctor*, showing a physician watching over a young boy in exactly the same way.

Third, my mother may have helped even more in getting me through that crisis, when she returned to my side in the hospital, which she'd left about an hour earlier, and gave me a real major-league baseball signed by Brooklyn Dodgers captain and shortstop Pee Wee Reese. She had gone to Ebbets Field and chased him down the gangway to the locker room. She knew that his signature on that baseball was the most tangible way to motivate me to want to be around for the Dodgers' next season.

Connected with these images there has always been the sense, especially strong during the rest of my growing up, that I owed something to others. My subsequent birthdays and life experiences have been gifts that would not have been mine to enjoy if the right people and techniques had not been in the right place at the right time.

From a strictly medical point of view, it was said that I survived only because of the recent availability of sulfanilamide, one of the first wonder drugs, which began to be used in the late 1930s. Sulfanilamide could not kill strep and other bacteria, but it could hold them in check and give the immune system a chance to rally.

I almost certainly would not have survived without the sulfanilamide. But I also think that I would not have survived without the benefit of mercy, hope, justice, and autonomy. My family, Dr. Cirillo and Dr. Shapiro, and the nurses and other hospital staff showed me mercy, instilled hope in me, and fought to give me a fair chance at a full life span. Insofar as autonomy is concerned, of course, I was not making decisions about my care at that age, and I was often left in the dark about exactly what was going on. But everyone gave me the sense that they were concerned about me as a unique person, and the doctors and other caregivers interacted with my parents in a way that showed respect for their autonomy and that of our family as a whole. In hindsight, I see the sulfanilamide not as something apart from all that, but as an instrument of mercy, hope, justice, and autonomy used in my care.

These experiences did not make me want to become a doctor, however. Until I was well along in college, I was sure that medicine was not for me. Following my parents' and my older brother's example, I wanted to do something useful, but I had no definite idea what that might be.

My parents were both born in 1898 in Brooklyn, New York, to immigrant Catholic families. Despite that common ground, they had to run away to get married when they were twenty years old. It was a scandalous mixed marriage, because my father was Irish and my mother was Italian. The Irish reached New York first, with the Italian wave of immigration starting a generation later. Bitter competition between the two groups on the lower rungs of the socioeconomic ladder persisted for a long time. Fortunately, after the wedding, everything seemed to work out amicably between my parents and the two sides of the extended family.

Neither of my parents had a true collegiate bachelor of arts degree obtained at the usual time. My mother had finished teacher-training school just before they eloped, which led her directly into a lifetime of teaching fifth grade. My father attended St. John's College and played shortstop on the baseball team before leaving to join the army during World War I. He then became a salesman and worked his way up at the Armour Company, which kept us with a steady supply of meats during the Depression. In 1927, they had their first child, my brother, Bill. He became a second father figure for me, even getting my name changed to Roger, from my parents' selection, Bruce, before I was born six years later. The reason why escapes me now, but I have never forgotten that he had a reason and that they all agreed to make the change. My parents plainly did not believe children should be seen and not heard, but might well have something interesting to say.

My mother's teaching was important to all of us, and we were proud that she was known as a good teacher. As the demography of the borough of Queens changed as more and more African Americans moved into it from Harlem, my mother remained very engaged in the same public school. I remember visiting her classroom while I was still in high school and appreciating that exactly half the class was white and half was black. This was about the time Jackie Robinson, followed by Roy Campanella, Don Newcombe, and Joe Black, were expanding the cultural horizons of baseball fans as players for the Dodgers. My mother was way ahead of most people in that regard. She wasn't preaching anything; she was just doing constructive things.

My father showed his respect for my mother as a working woman by doing the housework on Friday evenings and Saturdays, first by himself and then with the help of my brother and me, so she could get a day off. Eventually my father graduated to getting the day off too, and Bill and I did those chores. The valuable and enduring lesson for us, much as we disliked missing some schoolyard basketball games with our friends every week, was that my father took the lead in instituting this practice.

My father on the other hand was very frustrated about working only to make a living, as were many people during the Depression. He was outspoken about the problems he saw in our society, leading Bill and me to wish that he would do something besides rail at the world. I think we both vowed not to be in his position and to try to do something to make a difference. In fact, this was actually what he always tried to emphasize for us: to be as independent as possible while learning how to do something useful. Then one day the sons woke up to the fact that their father's attendance at night school five times a week for four years had been to learn chiropractic. He got his license, quit his job at Armour, opened up an office in Manhattan and one in our home, and lived a professional life analogous to the one he had been preaching. He was, from all we could determine, a very good chiropractor. Eventually, he taught me a number of things when I became a physician.

But as I said, I did not then want to enter medicine. My brother, however, was following the medical path. After attending the Merchant Marine Officers Training School and serving in the merchant marine from 1947 to 1949, Bill became a premed student at Cornell. He got a summer job at Columbia Presbyterian Medical Center, and one day he took me, then sixteen, to the observation room above an operating room to watch a fairly minor procedure. While the patient and doctor were still talking, a long needle was passed through the patient's abdominal skin, the fat underneath, and out through the skin again. What I suppose was local anesthetic was injected as the needle was withdrawn. That was as far as I got with that operation. I was relegated to sitting on the floor outside in the hall awaiting the return of full blood flow to my brain, while my brother watched the rest of the action. When it was over, I wished him well in his choice of careers, but supposed that I would be going some other way—any other way!

Bill earned a bachelor's degree in science at Cornell, decided against medical school, married, was called up to serve as a naval reserve officer during the Korean War, and returned to attend the University of Missouri School of Journalism, where he earned his master's degree. Until the day he died a few years back, he remained in most settings the most adept person I knew at placing himself psychologically in another person's shoes. I always thought he would have been a terrific physician because of the healing quality of his personality.

A series of other experiences confirmed my sense that I was not cut out for medicine. One of my schoolyard basketball friends was a skinny kid named John McDermott. When we met, he was trying to perfect a long one-handed shot, which had been introduced by the star of my high school team, Bob Cousy. John's family was poor in economic terms, but rich in other ways. A scholarship student successively at a Catholic high school in New York City, St. Francis College, and graduate school at Fordham University, during high school John became involved in a movement called Catholic Action, which originated with French worker-priests on the docks of Marseilles.

John assembled other kids who wanted to do something constructive for various activities. One activity I participated in was taking the subway on Sunday mornings from Queens to Bellevue Public Hospital in Manhattan, where we took patients to mass in the chapel and spent time with them and other patients afterward. Those bleak, cold, wintry mornings in a large, gray, impersonal environment with what seemed to me to be hopelessly suffering patients infected me with a sense of personal futility. I recognized the symbolic nature of our attempts to be helpful, but I didn't like any of it, and especially not the hospital atmosphere.

It was not until I went to Harvard College on a scholarship, majoring first in intellectual history and finally in English literature, that my thinking changed. What I understood of my motivations in life and my strengths and weaknesses seemed to point to medicine as the best way I could combine my religion and a sense of personal meaning with a line of work. I was fortunate enough to win admission to Harvard Medical School, and then I had some other luck that presented me with the kind of dilemma where, as Yogi Berra put it, "When you come to a fork in the road, take it."

Every year Harvard awards a graduating senior the Harvard Scholarship to spend a year at Cambridge University in England, living in the same rooms in Emmanuel College that John Harvard himself occupied as a student before he emigrated to America. To my surprise, the powers that be chose me. The dean of admissions at Harvard Medical School urged me not to take the scholarship, warning that I would have to reapply for admission with no guarantee of acceptance. That gave me pause, but in the end I decided to go, and I learned a lot from the experience of living in another country and being a student at Cambridge.

My one real task for the year was to organize the annual John Harvard Dinner, held in Emmanuel College's Long Gallery, which had been designed by Christopher Wren, the architect of St. Paul's Cathedral in London. This involved inviting a main speaker, and I thought immediately of T. S. Eliot. Eliot, who held a senior position in a distinguished British publishing firm, had attended college at Harvard and often returned there to speak. I wrote him while I was still at Harvard, and he was kind enough to exchange several letters with me before I got to England.

My correspondence with Eliot continued during my first months at Cambridge. Eventually, it became clear that he couldn't attend the John Harvard Dinner. But he did invite me to visit him, so one day I took the train down to London and went to see him in his office at Faber and Faber in Russell Square. I had just read his play *The Confidential Clerk*, about a character who works for a rich executive and serves to facilitate the lives of many of the other characters in the play. These characters invariably try to influence and control the clerk, but they all ultimately describe him as "somehow indifferent" and unwilling to take what is being offered to him. Finally, in love with the organ and music, he moves to the country as the organist for a parish church.

I kept trying to find out what Eliot meant about this personal indifference, but he was known not to answer questions from readers seeking such explanations and would not rise to the bait. Nonetheless, for a wonderful hour he sat at his desk beside a large window and chatted with me, drawing me out on my plans for the future. Looking variously at him and at the church steeple visible through the window, I shared my somewhat confused thoughts about my motives, strengths, and weaknesses, and the connections I saw between my religious instincts and service as a physician. As the conversation drew to a close, he seemed to connect my personal meanderings with his character's decision to become the organist in a village parish church and said, "The world needs good Catholic doctors!" He didn't need to say the corollary, which I knew to be "the world needs good doctors." I would swear that the church bells began to chime just then!

Bells or no bells and whatever he meant, what he said—and the simple fact that he invested time in someone he would never have contact with again—still speaks volumes to me about teaching without attempting to control and about some of the meaningful effects of even casual human interactions. The encounter also symbolizes for me the importance of bringing the full range of human and cultural values into the practice of medicine. This became more and more my focus after I graduated from Harvard Medical School in 1960 (fortunately, they did accept me again, when I duly reapplied) and embarked on the work as a physician, teacher, and administrator that I outlined in the introduction.

A Physician-Patient

In 1994, my life unexpectedly entered a totally new phase, when I received a computerized axial tomography (CAT or CT) scan of my mediastinum (the space behind the heart). Some months before, I had had a right middle-lobe bacterial pneumonia from which I recovered clinically, although the X-rays still showed some abnormality, prompting the CT scan. The scan revealed a large mass behind my heart that seemed to encircle the main stem bronchus leading to the lung. The list of possibilities included tumors frightening to anyone and called for prompt diagnosis, which meant a thoracotomy, biopsy, tissue diagnosis, and ultimately chemotherapy with three major metabolic poisons and a short course of prednisone. Five months of treatment was followed by diagnostic tests to ascertain whether I would fall among the three-quarters of patients who have a good outcome or among the one-quarter who face a more difficult future.

Thus, at sixty-one, and for the first time since age seven, I was confronting a serious illness that brought me into intense contact with the hospital and health care system as a patient rather than as a caregiver or administrator. This time I faced the possibility of fatal disease and the certain involvement with a systemic biologic poisoning that would, if all worked well and without complications, cause chronic illness for the duration of therapy and the ensuing recovery period. After it became clear that I was one of the lucky patients to have a remission, periodic CT and positron emission tomography (PET) scans kept reminding me that the illness would someday come back, unless I died of other causes in the meantime.

It was during this illness episode that I first had the experience of being a patient while at the same time being a physician. I saw many things through that special prism, both good and bad. I saw the efficiency, effectiveness, and compassion of the general internist, Dr. Bryan Arling, and of the oncologist he recommended, Dr Bruce Kressel, both of whom have taken care of me ever since. I appreciated how both of them consulted widely and carefully kept both my wife and me informed and involved. Dr. Arling even brought his partner to see me in the hospital as I was recovering from the thoracotomy and biopsy, so that his partner and I would know each other if he were ever called to treat me when Dr. Arling was elsewhere. I also learned how some of the various nurses and technicians had mastered the art of conveying a positive, even a healing, demeanor. These were all experiences in which mercy, hope, justice, and autonomy each had their due places.

But there were also experiences of a different sort. The first was the obvious discomfort one of the surgeons seemed to be experiencing in talking about what my biopsy showed. My bottom-line conclusion was that he identified closely with me both in age and as a physician and perhaps hadn't yet dealt adequately with the prospect of his own mortality (as indeed I had not). A variation on that theme occurred during a visit to see a pulmonary specialist, at the request of the primary care physician. The specialist left me getting dressed and went into the office next door. I heard his voice as he talked to my doctor on the phone. He thanked my doctor for sending me to him, said what a nice guy I was and how sad it was that such terrible diagnoses seem to come to nice people. I concluded that his error in leaving his door ajar was forgivable but that his interest in keeping his referral source alive and well was far greater than his compassion for me, the patient. I declined his offer of an office bronchoscopy before getting the needed definitive surgical biopsy, preferring to discuss that option with my own doctor. Doctors fall into such behaviors in dealing with patients, as they either struggle against the motivational disincentives of our perverse payment systems or game the systems to keep their practices viable and their incomes where they want them to be. I believe the trend among older physicians to recommend that their children not follow in their footsteps is related to their increasing battle to run their own independent businesses on a fee-for-service basis. Many of them are retiring as soon as possible, while others are moving toward salaried positions that insulate them from the business side of medical practice.

Our payment systems seem destined to be several, each with strengths and weaknesses in terms of incentives and disincentives for the delivery of ideal care. The best sign on the horizon is that more patients and medical professionals alike are examining their circumstances in terms of the incentives inherent in their insurances or payment systems. As time goes on, pressure from our health care system's gross inequity and rising costs, as well as mounting evidence of its overutilization by the affluent and underutilization by others, should help improve the quality and selection of the services rendered to everyone in the population.

Grateful for the Latest Breakthroughs

Four major impressions emerged from my 1994 illness. First and foremost was the constantly increasing sophistication of medical science and technology, delivered by an increasingly numerous and specialized health care team. I experienced some of the striking recent advances at that time in diagnosis and treatment, anesthesia, surgery, and cancer chemotherapy. Perhaps the most significant advance involved the CT scan and its role in finding the precise location of the initial lesion. Without that scan, my condition would likely have gone undetected for perhaps another year, while the lymphoma grew elsewhere and finally produced new symptoms.

Grateful for Human Support

The second, somewhat surprising finding was my realization of the enormous importance of human support from family and friends. The cards, letters, telephone calls, prayers, and positive sentiments all served to underscore and encourage my own and my family's commitment to do whatever was necessary for me to regain health. I have promised myself to never again be reluctant to extend such support to others for fear of intruding at such a personal time. It is, in fact, quite the opposite. Native Americans have long recognized the value of the tribe's support in the restoration of health; I now understand and appreciate that dimension far more intensely than ever before. I was not surprised by the attentions lavished upon me by my wife and daughters, but I was deeply gratified by them. Also, one of my nieces painstakingly made one thousand cut-out angels and sent them to me, which I found quite astonishing and welcome. In fact, it seems clear to me in retrospect that we caregivers, perhaps especially physicians, too often may grossly underestimate such support, focusing instead exclusively on the science and technology we know we can apply to a given medical problem.

Grateful for Retained Dignity

The third lesson learned (or relearned) through this illness in 1994 involves patient empowerment, independence, dignity, and psychological space. Harvard psychiatrist Leston Havens[1] has written that his therapeutic objective in psychotherapy is to create a relationship with his patient in which the two can figuratively occupy "the same space" and meaningfully interact, while feeling no need to either invade or be invaded by the other. Implicit in this simple approach is an enormous respect for the dignity and selfhood of the other. Attention to this need is terribly important when patients are physically sick and threatened with potentially fatal diseases. Being treated with respect by all the important players during my illness helped me handle the situation in general and cope with the many daily decisions. My caregivers also were assiduous in attempting to impart the best information and advice that they could, and then in encouraging me to make the decisions and to set the course. In those instances when there really was no alternative to their professional judgments, they were careful to inform me and to provide an opportunity for me to react.

Combining this sort of approach with the overwhelming support of family and friends, the skills of health professionals, and our advanced technology offers the best potential for effective interventions on behalf of the patient. There is no doubt in my mind that the lines begin to blur between the individuals who participate in this network of patient support and the health care institutions through which much of the work is carried out. The interface between individual caregivers and institutions can be highly constructive from the patient's point of view, or it can be quite the opposite. Both extremes occur, as do all the possibilities in between. Identifying and improving those less than optimal possibilities define the agenda for the health care professional team and system in the ongoing attempt to provide technically competent and humane care. That agenda increasingly requires direct input from the patient, whenever possible, at the key decision points. Most doctors in my experience seem to know this and are acting in that vein. Some health care institutions are bringing patients onto their committees and task forces. I believe more and more patients will welcome that approach and, in fact, demand it.

The Gift of Mercy

When I finally digested my feelings and thoughts about my illness in 1994, I wrote a book entitled *The Quest for Mercy*. I drew a good deal on what I learned from reading some of the writings of Marcus Borg, a prominent New Testament scholar. Discussing Jesus's call that we treat others with compassion, Borg explains that the word Jesus used for compassion—literally, "wombness" in Hebrew—refers to a mother's encircling support and concern for her child. Over two millennia, the word "wombness" has become the word "mercy."

This rich meaning of mercy first clicked for me when I was rereading a passage of Thomas Merton's about the words that all novitiates say upon entering the Trappist order of monks. Merton himself had uttered these words when he began his long, complex, and now very public journey into the life of the spirit. To the ritual question, "What do you ask?" Merton gave the ritual answer, "I ask for the mercy of God and of the order." Somehow, for me those ritual words would have been more spiritually activating if they had been "I ask for the encircling concern and support of God and of the order."

Thanks to Borg's explanation of how "wombness" became "compassion" or "mercy," I made a new connection regarding patients and the role that the health care system plays in our society. He also provided some new words with which to communicate with patients in different settings. When gravely ill, suddenly disabled, or near death, even the most independent and strong among us seek the mercy (or the encircling concern and support) of our society through our family and friends, and from our individual caregivers and organized health care delivery systems. Everyone may need such mercy or compassion one day. Yet compassion requires time. With health care time rationed in the interest of economy, as it is these days, Americans could organize and administrate themselves right out of compassion.

For thousands of years, cultures have assigned high status and special designations to healers and leaned heavily on their compassionate efforts. It would be a tragedy, just when we have so many effective scientific therapies at hand, for policy makers to negotiate away the element of compassion, leaving this crucial dimension of healing solely to nonscientific healers or to no one. In other words, we scientifically trained healers must develop and sustain health care that shows mercy when people most need it—and that is when they are suffering!

One of my conclusions in that book was as follows:

Clearly, in the postmodern world, the concept of the solo physician is a thing of the past and must be extended to include many other health team members. Clearly too this foundation is not fully consistent with the financial arrangements, perverse incentives and bureaucracy inherent in our current situation. My own illness has underscored my personal commitment to work toward a health care reform that preserves the special therapeutic bond between the health professionals and the sufferer, a bond that is central to the seeking of mercy, one to another! I cannot escape the notion that the extent to which we succeed in maintaining the humanity of our health care system should be an important measure of the quality of our twenty-first century civilization. For me, then the name of the game is, indeed, mercy!"[2]

What I have experienced since then has only strengthened that conclusion. To return to Merton, if I had been asked by anyone as a patient with a life-threatening disease, "What do you ask?" my answer would have been that I was asking society for mercy in extending to me, through its health professionals, its institutions, my family, and loved ones the requisite help to deal with the difficult matters at hand, because I could not do it alone. Whether the helpers are office colleagues or hospital specialists, the sufferer needs their merciful support. At the core must be a latticework of morally accountable, concerned health professionals. Their time-honored commitment to the patient's welfare remains central to our system of health care, which of late shows signs of being devoured by perverse financial arrangements, incentives, and health system structures much as termites damage a house from within.

Facing Life-Threatening Illness Again

In the summer of 2007, the mixed-cell lymphoma recurred. Trying to make sense of a new set of illness experiences, and almost by serendipity, I discovered two records written by physicians. They had each also been stricken suddenly with a potentially fatal disease while asymptomatic and happily working away. The first is a brief account by John C. Vander Woude,[3] a young cardiothoracic surgery resident, who was discovered on routine examination to have a malignant lymphoma. Because he was about thirty years old and close to his most productive professional years, his disease posed a completely different threat to him and his young family than the one I faced. But his experience with the sudden transition from being a high-powered operative, controlling the levers of the hospital, to a passive recipient of orders was similar to mine. It enhanced his understanding, as it did mine, of what the patient goes through at the hands of a health care team and within the sometimes grinding gears of the hospital and overall health care system. For example, as a patient needing his blood drawn at the chemistry lab, he had to wait in line as a supplicant in a setting he used to dominate as a house physician. I'm sure he found this a valuable lesson in humility, as it was for me.

Perhaps the most striking description of what a sensitive physician-turned-patient can learn and consequently can teach the rest of us has been written by Fitzhugh Mullan.[4] A routine chest X-ray revealed that this young physician had a tumor. In Mullan's case, the problem was much more severe than mine, the diagnostic process was far more complicated and life-threatening, the course in the hospital and treatment to eventual recovery much more prolonged, and the ordeal far more anxiety producing and trying for his family and professional life. A vignette from Mullan's story leads into one of the major points I wish to make from my own experience.

After an extraordinarily long, grueling, and heart-rending

struggle with cancer treatment and rehabilitation, Mullan was ready for discharge from the hospital's protective environment to what now seemed to him a threatening and strange outside world. On that day of discharge he felt, perhaps for the first time, a strong desire to take his own life. Grappling with his feelings, he let the hospital staff know that he needed some help. Shortly, a staff psychiatrist arrived. After listening briefly to the distraught patient, the psychiatrist asked, "Do you want me to hold you?" Those seven words turned the entire situation around. The reader of Mullan's book leaves the scene with the vision of two grown men embracing: one giving of his strength to the other—embattled, scared, and suffering—the power to continue the struggle toward a return to well-being.

This striking story brought home what I have often observed in a less dramatic fashion, namely, the capacity of specialists who do not have frequent or continuing deep encounters with a patient to say or do the right thing at just the right time to hasten the march to recovery. Over the years, I have encountered some of the reverse as well. But the lesson remains that both the generalist and the specialist have enormous opportunities to influence the course of the patient's treatment, in ways that flow from emotional intelligence and compassion as well as professional and technical expertise.

Five Lessons from My Last Illness

LESSON 1. The discovery of an unexpected posttraumatic syndrome came to my attention when I woke up to begin another new day, about two months after my last treatment and my last finally normal PET scan. After completing the third round of monthly weeklong hospital treatments with five different chemotherapeutic agents, the plan was to get a PET scan before taking a single treatment with Zevalin. Zevalin was one of a couple of very promising new agents designed to selectively seek out and attach to malignant lymphoma cells, thus allowing an attached radioactive substance to destroy these marked cancerous cells one at a time. This last treatment was one of two possibilities presented to me, the other being massive doses of chemotherapeutics, after storing some of my own bone marrow and returning it sometime after the toxic levels of chemotherapy had diminished. This approach is known to be successful in many people if they survive the treatment itself. That choice was up to me as the patient. We had decided on the Zevalin route if possible.

As I was preparing to leave the hospital after the third round of treatment, I felt dizzy and unable to stand to get dressed. I was in short order found to have a gram-negative septicemia that, as a former infectious disease specialist, I recognized as a critical and often fatal syndrome. After two more harrowing weeks in intensive care and in surgery for a cholecystectomy (the gall bladder was deemed to be the most likely source of the E. coli that caused the septicemia), I was discharged a lot thinner but with Zevalin the only prudent treatment option left for me. Happily, the PET scan turned out well and I got my radioactive infusion without side effects or untoward reactions. Parenthetically, the charge for the Zevalin treatment was $80,000.

I go into this detail because the reader needs to know it in order to make better sense of the traumatic nature of the illness and that if I had developed any of the usual stress-related symptoms, it would not have surprised my doctors. But that didn't happen. Except for the anticipated weakness and the slow and gradual recovery period, I felt happy enough to be alive even in the face of my low energy level. Then, in early December, just two months after the Zevalin treatment, I woke up and got out of bed feeling normal; not special, just normal! Feeling normal was something I hadn't experienced for at least six months, and I decided that it would soon go away, probably by the time I slowly got downstairs. But within minutes, I realized the return of normalcy wasn't going away. That was special, very special.

In fact, I experienced euphoria centered in my perceived good fortune to have somehow been granted normalcy again for a few hours or maybe some days or maybe even longer. But for whatever the time, it was clear that I was and have remained grateful for every moment of life so far! Frankly, I was reticent to tell anyone but my wife, who is also my best friend, because I didn't understand it and couldn't put a name to it. My first thought as a scientifically trained physician was that my recovery had reached a biochemical stage at which some metabolic pathways were switched on that had been in limbo for some months, and that may in fact be the case. Then I came upon Jennifer Michael Hecht's recent book, *The Happiness Myth*,[5] in which she recounts how some postcancer patients, encountering death and yet not dying, experienced "Post-Traumatic Bliss"! It rang a bell and allowed me a venue through which to introduce the subject to colleagues and others, but no one seemed to know anything about it.

Just at that time, I was asked to write a two-hundred-word opinion piece for a medical journal. I decided to test the editor's courage by describing my own experience with posttraumatic bliss. The concerns I had that people would think this was a harebrained idea were erased by the extraordinary responses from doctors, nurses, and psychologists. Many of them shared their stories of encounters with life-changing illness episodes that seem to have left their marks for years.[6]

A striking recent example of making something out of available time when facing serious illness and the possibility of death has been the course chosen by Professor Randy Pausch of Carnegie Mellon University. Pausch, in his forties, with a wife and three small children, was diagnosed with inoperable and untreatable pancreatic cancer in 2007. In September of that year, he gave a universitywide lecture he entitled "The Last Lecture."[7] His subject was his new diagnosis and how he intended to deal with the time he had left. He dedicated his lecture to his wife and children and the rest of his life to providing the latter with enough memories of their dad to last a lifetime. He died in the summer of 2008, having achieved national and international acclaim for a book based on his lecture. He had literally taught millions of readers invaluable lessons about life and the importance of making the most of every day. His example was his dedication to a superordinate goal, in his case his family.

Another phenomenal example of what I am talking about is the very moving speech made at the Democratic National Convention by Senator Ted Kennedy in Denver, Colorado, on August 25, 2008. Under active treatment for a malignant brain tumor, his prognosis was at best guarded and his therapy stripped him of much of his energy. Against the advice of his doctors and his wife, he flew to Denver to speak at the convention. He promised that the dream of social justice and universal health care was still alive and that he fully intended to be in the Senate in January 2009 to help see those initiatives through to fruition. Clearly, whatever one thinks of his politics, here was a person confronting his own grave circumstances by throwing himself fully into an effort to benefit others—a superordinate goal, the pursuit of which surely made his remaining days more meaningful, even if it didn't extend them.

For the rest of us who cannot hope to have such dramatic impact on the public, I believe the lesson is the same as it was for Pausch and Kennedy. Even in some of the darkest times, I found that I was happiest when I was able to focus on the other person rather than myself. That is the lesson of holocaust survivor and existential psychiatrist Viktor Frankl's classic *The Search for Meaning*: that finding meaning in our lives and days is our ultimate purpose.[8,9]

During his last trip to America in the mid-1990s, when he was nearly ninety years old, Viktor Frankl spoke at the University of Texas

Health Science Center at Houston, where I was then president. The reason for inviting him to speak was that the dean of our school of nursing, Pat Starck, had received her PhD for her work in applying Frankl's philosophy to severely handicapped patients and debilitating illnesses in general. She was chosen for her position over other excellent candidates precisely because of that background.

The audience to hear Frankl not only completely filled every seat in the largest lecture hall in the Texas Medical Center, wheel chairs and litters carrying dozens of paraplegics and quadriplegics also lined the aisles. I shall not forget his talk that day, particularly his story of a patient who could only write with a pencil in her mouth. Each day she constructed a note of encouragement to someone whose misfortune she discovered through her nurse's daily reading of the newspaper. This activity gave her a reason for, and satisfaction in, living.

LESSON 2. The illness experience itself can be a time of significant personal growth. I learned, for example, the extent to which my illness can affect others, especially within the circle of family and close friends. Clearly, Randy Pausch and Ted Kennedy have left an amazing set of examples and lessons for those who are influenced by them. According to an interesting book written by David Rieff,[10] author Susan Sontag's son, Sontag was dedicated to searching for the cure for her cancer and never talked about the gravity of her diagnosis or her impending death with him. Hers was another way.

Francis Moore, the brilliant and charismatic surgeon, shocked many when one evening, late in his life, he left the family dinner table and, as was his habit, went to his office upstairs—only this evening instead of studying and writing, he took out his revolver and blew his brains out. Michael DeBakey, another surgical genius, lived into his nineties, when he was stricken with a leaking aortic aneurysm. Although he resisted approving for himself the dramatic surgical treatment that he had invented and which had saved so many younger persons, the hospital ethics committee approved the surgery when he became unresponsive. He recovered and resumed his active international professional life until dying of natural causes a year or so thereafter.

When the end seems near, how does one handle it? Faced with the relentless progress of Parkinson's disease and an associated form of dementia, George Bernier, one of my best friends and a medical school classmate, found a way, with his wife and family, to stay the course until the end. George was the quintessential physician triple-threat: a fine clinician, an excellent researcher, and an absolutely superb teacher and role model. His wife, Mary Jane, established herself as his equal in these three dimensions as a nurse. Thus it shouldn't be surprising that one of them chose to live the end of his life in a way that could teach by example. When the time came, George understood that it was best for him to move into the nearby nursing home, uttering not a word of complaint about the move. Having served as dean of two major American medical schools, he spent his last weeks of life making daily visits to the other nursing home patients, with a stethoscope draped around his neck, probably believing that he was still a physician, until he passed away quietly in his sleep one night.

Let Mary Jane fill in some details in her own words:

George's diagnosis was of a Parkinson's-related form of dementia, which demonstrates wide swings of confusion and periods of lucidity. That part made his illness especially cruel because there were moments when he was still with me and understanding of what was happening . . . of his loss of self. It was the social worker at Belmont Manor who suggested we do things to reinforce George's role as a physician. This was discussed at a multidisciplinary meeting (absent the MD) and it was Elizabeth (our physician daughter) who took her stethoscope out of her bag to give to George. I developed a special 'chart' for him that looked like all the other patient charts and he could come to the desk and ask for his chart. I filled it with reprints of his publications, the current issue of the *New England Journal of Medicine*, and notepaper. When I collected his belongings on the morning of his death, I went into the activity room and his chart was open on the table. I loved the idea that he was looking at that the evening before he died and that his stethoscope was in his hand. The value of multidisciplinary approaches to health care was a lived experience for me.

I have personally known all the people mentioned above, except for Randy Pausch and Susan Sontag. In general, I find that I am most often influenced by how those I know personally handle life's biggest challenges. I guess it is another way that those we know and respect can continue to influence us and why we all remain important to those who know us.

Illness episodes provide opportunities for people to consider the deepest personal issues of life and death. As E. B. White[11] used to claim that "loneliness and privacy" were the gifts New York City provided its denizens, it is well to consider that loneliness and privacy may be important pieces of the puzzle of care and of dealing with serious illness. As a New Yorker, I connect with White's observation about the value of sometimes being able to be alone in the crowd. The time to consider the balance between hope and reality for the patient's situation needs to be respected for the patient and the family and friends.

The opportunity to look at the bright side of the cloud of suffering allows some people to find "strength in broken places," as Hemingway said. It is the subject of an important recent book of that title by Richard Cohen.[12] Cohen found several individuals with incurable chronic diseases. His descriptions of their journeys, including his reflections on his own multiple sclerosis, bring the reader into closer connection with and appreciation for their difficult and extraordinary lives.

LESSON 3: If I can get expensive and effective treatment at age seventy-five, shouldn't every American? It wasn't long ago that ethicist Dan Callahan, formerly the director of the Hastings Center, whom I know and respect, proposed that at some point around the age of seventy-five and thereafter, people should no longer be given dramatic and expensive interventions, which in most instances will do little to usefully extend quality life years. When I was sixty-one, my employer-based health insurance paid for most of the high cost of the complex professional and pharmaceutical interventions I needed, which successfully provided me with a full remission of disease for fourteen years. We never thought I was totally free of malignant cells and expected that if I lived long enough, the disease would reappear. Eleven years later, I retired in continuing good health and switched to Medicare as my health insurer. I had both parts A and B from the outset and shortly thereafter purchased parts C and D, the former being "gap" insurance and the latter pharmaceutical coverage. Parts C and D cost around $170 a month.

Thus, when my illness did return with a vengeance, the oncologist was able to treat me as I detailed earlier. I cannot tell you how grateful my family and I are for the chemotherapeutic combinations and new drug developments of the past two decades. There are no guarantees, of course, but my own treatment has brought me back to where I am trying to contribute to my family and to do what I can to help our nation get over the hill that separates us from deciding to implement a system (or systems) to make health insurance available for every American. I became even more convinced when I saw the bills come in for my care: $200,000 total, $80,000 of which was for the Zevalin (completely covered at that time by Medicare). With all my various insurances, we paid less than 5 percent of the cost out of pocket. Health insurance gave me my life back; without it I would have been loath to be treated. Almost 50 million uninsured citizens, and a larger number who are drastically underinsured, face the threat of personal bankruptcy from health care costs, however. This surely raises the concept of health care as a right for all Americans to the level of a moral imperative.

There is no doubt that providing financial access to care for all Americans raises the question of rationing, which in turn leads most people to a consideration of creating a reasonable and acceptable list of services to be made universally available. In my view, we must create a public commission to determine which services are effective enough to be made available to everyone. Newer treatments not yet proven to be of value may be either left to be researched through publicly or privately supported clinical trials, or provided to people willing to pay for them through a private insurance supplement or their own private resources. It used to be that the poor were the subpopulation most likely to get new unproven treatments. In the current and next era, the pendulum for such experimental and potentially innovative treatments seems likely to swing toward the more affluent subpopulation. We may therefore be tending to experiment on the rich. We cannot give everyone everything that looks promising, but we can guarantee everyone a health insurance program that gives access to technologies, treatments, and protocols shown to be effective and basic to health.

The dirty little secret explaining why the health care industry opposes extensive health care reform is that much of its profit comes from treatments that are either ineffective, of uncertain effectiveness, or vastly and wastefully overutilized.

LESSON 4: After reflecting more fully upon my time as a physician-turned-patient, I saw what the greatest advantage was for me, over those without significant insider health care experience. Not only was I accepted as a member of my own health care team, but I also served as the de facto analogue to the chair of a company's board of directors. The doctors and nurses were the chief executives. I realized especially after it was all over that my friends and professional contacts, only an email away in most instances, allowed me and particularly my family the comfort of knowing that whatever steps, chances, and attendant risks we were taking or planning were sensible. My own doctor's judgments and those of the myriad specialists operating within his orbit were supported by the second opinions he obtained, as well as by those I secured through direct and email contacts.

There are so many things one doesn't understand and often doesn't remember, or is hesitant to bring up in the hurly-burly of ongoing patient care, that in complex situations it is simply impossible for the doctor or nurse to cover everything one wants to know. However, with the rapid development of information technology, including social networking among specific patient disease groups and advanced publicly available medical information sources, we are moving toward the more fully educated patient—a patient who can in fact become the chair of the board of a personal health care company. The challenge is how to help more patients get to the point where they can comfortably fill that position in a constructive and productive manner, without becoming medical micromanagers.

LESSON 5: Background material about the environment in which modern personal health care and its clinicians and administrators should function must be developed and provided to all patients. I have spent much of my professional academic life attempting to identify, describe, and communicate to health professionals in training the factors that will contribute to effective, humane health promotion, disease treatment, and chronic care and rehabilitation.

These issues include human values and ethics; pain and suffering;

communication; the placebo effect and the trusting relationship; healing environments; cultural diversity; disparities in health status; the distribution of health care services; rationing; covenantal relationships in the health professions; and how to envision an optimal future for health care delivery in the United States. Over the past several decades, there has been a growing trend to incorporate these broader, often nonscientific subjects in medical training. Clearly, giving young doctors, dentists, and nurses a significant grounding in these matters will be increasingly crucial to effective patient- and population-centered health care.

In like manner, patients must have access to more resources, including electronic health records, if they are to function as board chairs in their own health care decisions. Since my recovery, I have come to understand more clearly what I learned during more or less extended sojourns as a "full-time patient." I wish I had consciously known some of these things when I was a practicing clinician. I have concluded that these lessons might be valuable not only to other physicians, nurses, and other caregivers but, more important, to people who are or will be patients: people who must participate in the management of their own serious, potentially fatal acute and chronic diseases.

From 1940 to 1994 to 2007, when my three encounters with life-threatening illness occurred, the complexity and cost of all aspects of the health care system have increased at an accelerating rate. The treatments possible, the numbers and categories of health professionals needed to deliver them, and the bureaucracy that administers everything have grown to the point where health care has become America's largest industry—and where reforming the system has become both a political nightmare and an urgent practical necessity. Let's take a closer look at what that entails for both patients and their caregivers.

Chapter 2

Healing with Technology and with Words, Art, and the Senses

Medicine: "The Silent Art" No Longer!

About twenty-five hundred years ago, the Greek physician Hippocrates and his followers insisted that medicine move away from the soothsayers, the spell casters, the shamans, and the verbal magicians who used language as their healing instrument. Doctors in the Hippocratic tradition were to become doers: people of tangible actions seeking to find and employ new and better methods of intervening in the disease processes afflicting their patients. Talking, as curative, had no place in Hippocratic medicine, whereupon medicine became known as "the silent art."[1] This trend has continued, defining medicine as a science and practice based on nature, observation, reasoning, and action—and not on words.

For most of the last two and a half millennia, however, biomedical science advanced so slowly that the therapeutic value of the silent art was more promise than fact. What nonverbal tools doctors had usually didn't work or were downright harmful. Words still constituted most of what doctors could use to ameliorate suffering. They personally stood by their patients, watching them through their illnesses and advising their families. They offered human support.

The physician's ability to do more than set broken bones and sit with a patient through a fever began to change dramatically with the birth of modern biology and chemistry in the late eighteenth century. Among other developments during that time, Edward Jenner established that it was possible to vaccinate against smallpox and the discovery of oxygen exploded the theory that burning something up in a fire released the mysterious element phlogiston. The nineteenth and early twentieth centuries saw medicine transformed, often against the medical establishment's stiff resistance, by the gradual acceptance of vaccination; discoveries about microbes and the importance of hand washing; Pasteur's demonstration of how "pasteurization" prevented bovine tuberculosis transmission to humans; the Curies' development of the X-ray; and important advances in sanitation and other public health measures.

In the first half of the twentieth century, the ongoing search for the "magic bullet" spearheaded by the German chemical industry gave birth to sulfanilamide, perhaps the first effective antimicrobial. Although it couldn't kill them, sulfanilamide kept microbes from proliferating to a degree that human host defenses became much more effective. It played a role in my recovery from double pneumonia as a seven-year-old in 1940.

In 1928, Alexander Fleming was checking some Petri dishes in which he had been growing staphylococcus bacteria when he noticed a mold was killing the staph in one dish. He identified his serendipitous discovery as *Penicillium notatum*. However, it was not until World War II that the Oxford University team of Walter Florey, Ernst Chain, and Norman Heatley demonstrated penicillin's value in fighting against infections. The magic bullet seemed to have been found at last.

During the 1960s, I was asked to study the laboratory effectiveness of two synthetic penicillins. The pharmaceutical company sponsoring the experiment wanted to know the potential for mixing them together in a form capable of being taken by mouth and used against several classes of bacteria, including methicillin-resistant staph. A routine study showed that mixing the two antibiotics did not reduce either's effect and did make them useful against a much broader range of infections. In reporting the findings in a journal article, however, I recommended against combining the antibiotics for fear of developing superresistant bugs. The science was beginning to shift our search from a single magic bullet to a series of medicines with distinct but smaller ranges of effectiveness.

The past sixty years have brought even more dramatic changes to the practice of medicine. New medical technologies and pharmaceuticals have tumbled out of science laboratories and industrial development enterprises in an increasing cascade. Doctors now have tools at their disposal to diagnose and treat a myriad of once hopeless conditions. Spectacular new noninvasive scanning devices provide unbelievably detailed analyses of physical abnormalities without even requiring the patient to speak to the doctor. Although it must be pointed out that Freud brought talking and listening back to the treatment of mental illness, talk therapy was more or less restricted to psychiatry. Paradoxically, the growing success of psychoactive drug therapy has meant that now more and more psychiatrists are busy directing drug therapy, while they leave the talking part of psychotherapy to psychologists. One school of thought even argues that traditional psychoanalysis should be recognized more for its contributions to the humanities and arts than its therapeutic value.[2]

The idea that modern medicine and medical technology have drastically improved our lives is widely accepted, even though these same advances seem at times to be overly mechanistic, impersonal, expensive, and frightening. One might even contend that the silent art should become even more silent, because it is simply not cost effective for today's expensively educated, technocratic physicians to indulge in the human support function. However, an alternative argument can be made. It is based in part upon the growing body of scientific evidence regarding the biochemical impact of highly charged verbal communication. Because of what we have begun to learn (or relearn) about the link between language and healing, physicians are increasingly joining nurses, social workers, and the more patient-centered institutions in exploiting the therapeutic power of their own words and those of their clinical teammates.

The Power of Words

Modern advances in neurochemistry and the brain sciences have revealed many connections between emotional states and the production or secretion of certain hormones or other chemicals. For example, brain endorphins are the body's own morphinelike substances, the production or secretion of which is influenced by a variety of external factors. A large body of research has developed on depression, stress, and negative emotions and their corresponding negative impacts on immune function. It thus becomes possible to envision how clinicians could use words as therapy, if they only knew how to affect the patient's emotional state in a predictable, appropriate manner.

Many physicians have developed their capacity to use words as therapy through personal observation and trial and error. One of the most influential commentators on this area of treatment was a layman, Norman Cousins, who learned from his own serious illnesses and then wrote compellingly about what he learned. In his bestselling book *The Anatomy of an Illness*,[3] Cousins describes how his cardiologist, Dr. Bernie Lown, told him that the most important therapeutic first step for a heart attack victim was for the doctor to meet the patient in the emergency room and say that everything was under control and that he or she would be all right. When he was able to do this, Dr. Lown seldom had to give the traditional shot of morphine to the patient. Reassuring words founded on a relationship of trust were effective enough therapy on their own.

In a path-breaking study, James Kennell and his colleagues[4] at Baylor College of Medicine and the Jefferson Davis Hospital in Houston found a similar dynamic at work in the case of women giving birth while accompanied by a supportive female companion called a "doula," a term derived from an ancient Greek word for a female servant. The doulas in the study were women who had themselves experienced normal vaginal deliveries with good outcomes, who were comfortable with patients and staff from all backgrounds, and who had gone through a brief training period during which they became familiar with hospital labor and delivery procedures. In a randomly controlled trial, the researchers found that the continuous presence of a doula during labor and delivery significantly reduced the rate of cesarean section deliveries (from 18% to 8%), the use of epidural anesthesia (from 55.3% to 7.8%), and the use of oxytocin to augment labor (from 43.6% to 17%). Doula support also was associated with a reduction in the duration of labor and in the rates of prolonged infant hospitalizations and maternal fevers.

The mechanisms by which doula support influences these various positive outcomes are not fully understood. Studies in animals and humans have pointed to a link between acute maternal anxiety and disturbances in the progress in normal labor. It seems likely that a doula can decrease maternal anxiety by her interactions with the laboring woman, her constant presence, physical touch, reassurance, explanations, and anticipatory guidance. All this in turn helps the laboring woman feel safer and calmer, so that labor can proceed as naturally and smoothly as possible. Kennell and colleagues suggested that the addition of doulas to obstetrical care teams for all laboring women would reduce medical care costs. Indeed, in the intervening two decades since this study was published, the doula concept has been widely adopted in America and worldwide, providing dramatic improvements in patient care and significant reductions in hospital and medical costs. An important observation to note here is that these extraordinary benefits derive totally from lay persons and the prudence of the care-giving organization in hiring them.

Norman Cousins, already well known as an editor and literary critic, turned his talents toward health and medical care after being diagnosed with heart disease and arthritis. Coming to believe that positive feelings can produce therapeutic gains by inducing internal chemical changes, he took the opportunity of his own illness to experiment firsthand with his ideas about emotions and health. One of his experiments involved watching humorous television programs and movies, like *Candid Camera* and Marx Brothers comedies. He reported, "It worked! I made the joyous discovery that ten minutes of genuine belly laughter has an anesthetic effect and would give me at least two hours of pain-free sleep."[5]

Writing forty years ago, Cousins also noted the curious slant of "psychobiological" research toward the study of negative emotions and their effects on health:

Increasingly, in the medical press, articles are being published about the high cost of negative emotions. Cancer, in particular, has been connected to intensive states of grief or anger or fear. It makes little sense to suppose that emotions exact only penalties and confer no benefits. At any rate, long before my own illness, I became convinced that creativity, the will to live, hope, faith, and love have biochemical significance and contribute strongly to healing and well-being. The positive emotions are life-giving experiences."[6]

Only in recent years has scientific attention to positive emotions and attitudes matched Cousins's prescient words. The evidence so far does not support any firm conclusions, but it is clear that belief and emotion can play powerful roles in such little understood but unquestioned phenomena like the placebo effect.

In this regard, another of Cousin's major observations had to do with the importance of positive doctor-patient interaction. He believed that one of the physician's primary responsibilities is to engage the patient's own capacity to mobilize the forces of mind and body to fight disease. Positive doctor-patient interaction need not consume a great deal of time. Studies show that hospitalized patients perceive the same one- or two-minute visit from their doctor to be much longer in duration if the doctor sits down at the bedside rather than stands in the doorway. As Cousins noted, empathy is an essential ingredient in a healing relationship. Coming into the patient's room and sitting at the bedside brings the doctor physically closer to what it means to be bedridden, all the more so if this includes a gentle, reassuring touch. Empathy thus can be expressed in many symbolic yet tangible ways.

My own observations as both a patient and physician are that caregivers are increasingly implementing Cousins's implicit recommendations. Such signs of empathy include not only the doctor's sitting down sometimes, but also the growing practice of allowing trained dogs to visit a patient ward or outpatient area; the utilization of music and the visual arts, particularly in pediatric environments; and efforts to develop a welcoming environment for close family and visitors. For example, during my hospitalization in 2007, my good friend Yosaif August sent me one of the award-winning hospital-bed curtains he had designed. When drawn around my bed, the curtain opened up to show a wonderful picture of a mountain stream and meadow. Everyone liked it so much, I soon reversed it so that the picture faced the doorway. I can't prove it, but I think the hospital staff came in more frequently after that, showing how an empathetic connection benefits both patients and caregivers alike. (The curtains, which display photomurals of nature scenes and have been tested in hospital studies, are available through Yosaif's company, Bedscapes/Healing Environments, www.bedscapes.com).

In *Making Contact: Uses of Language in Psychotherapy*, psychiatrist Leston Havens describes how the therapist may use words, facial expressions, and body language to convey empathy to the patient. In 1959, Dr. Havens instructed me and a few other medical students as we rotated through a month on a psychiatric ward. I have never forgotten his almost magical capacity to interview patients he'd never met before, engaging them constructively while extracting psychologically relevant information. When I came across his book years later, his commentary rang true to my recollections. He refers to language as "the engineering structure necessary to translate passion [i.e., a deep sense of caring] into what is clinically effective." Using empathy in healing opens new doors for therapists as well, by increasing their sensitivity to the feelings and needs of others. Havens goes on, "To find another, you must enter that person's world. The empathic visitor then discovers what he has taken for granted in his own world: that it is a world of particular time and space." [7]

Related to understanding how patients feel is understanding what patients think about their illness and how their treatment ought to proceed. Here, Norman Cousins, our quintessential patient representative, and an increasing number of leading clinicians who care deeply about helping patients heal themselves agree: shared decision making is another important endeavor in which good communication can exert a therapeutic impetus. In shared decision making between doctors and their patients, effective communication both enhances a patient's understanding of his or her condition and reinforces the sense of self-determination. Both these factors can reduce fear and depression and their negative physiological correlates. Cousins wrote, "If I had to guess, I would say that the principal contribution made by my doctor to the taming, and possibly the conquest, of my illness was that he encouraged me to believe I was a respected partner with him in the total undertaking."[8] Although these ideas were not unfamiliar to some of history's greatest clinicians, Cousins's writings made a remarkable contribution to medicine. He brought these ideas to many other patients and would-be patients and heightened the awareness of the health professions in general.

Experienced clinicians increasingly believe that participation in the clinical decision-making process is the most important element in determining the quality of the doctor-patient relationship.[9] The exceptional patient wants to share responsibility for his treatment, and doctors who encourage this attitude can help all their patients heal faster. The growing trend toward using words as therapy should help physicians divest themselves of that aspect of our Hippocratic heritage that devalues words as restorative tools. It should enhance effective collaboration with nurses and psychologists, whose professional cultures have long emphasized such emotional support in patient relations. Caregivers should seek to help all patients participate in decision making, and patients should not be shy about asking caregivers to do so.

Modern Medicine and the Word

Despite growing signs of improvement in this area, too few medical practitioners actively seek to heal with their words. They seem not to realize that words can be therapeutic or toxic. Many physicians have benefitted from teachers who were exceptional role models of expressing empathy to patients in word and deed. But the medical school experience as a whole tends to highlight scans and X-rays, blood tests, surgical interventions, hormones, drugs, and chemotherapy as effective diagnostic and therapeutic interventions and to minimize the value of talk. It also soon becomes clear to everyone that the physician who is not a psychiatrist gets little financial remuneration for talking with patients.

The result is that physicians are all too often uncomfortable with words and fail to see their usefulness in the fight against a tangible disease. Yet at some level most doctors realize that their words can have tremendous impact on at least some patients; it's just not a scientific thing. This is disquieting in part because even as the profession seems to be ever more effective in utilizing science and technology, much of the public has turned to nonscience-based healers to satisfy perceived gaps in their personal health care. Although physicians retain much of their traditional status in our society, they also strike many people as somewhat inhumane, mechanistically oriented, and materialistic.

Physician, medical scientist, and acclaimed author Dr. Lewis Thomas, whom I think of as an unofficial poet laureate of modern biology, deplored the modern hospital's incompatibility with the therapy of the word.

> Today, with the advance of medicine's various complicated new technologies, the ward rounds now at the foot of the bed, the drawing of blood samples for automated assessment of every known (or suggested) biochemical abnormality, the rolling of wheelchairs and litters down through the corridors to the x-ray department, there is less time for talking. The longest and most personal conversations held with hospital patients when they come to the hospital are discussions of finances and insurance, engaged in by personnel trained in accountancy, whose scientific instruments are the computers."[10]

These observations from the early 1990s still ring true, sad to say, but there have been significant improvements in many hospital environments. In addition to the movement toward single rooms for patients and a variety of aesthetic and creature comfort amenities, some hospital administrators and leaders have given their employees training in customer-oriented behavior and satisfaction. Progress in many aspects of patient-centered care is visible in our health care institutions, including that flowing from the concerted efforts to monitor and improve the quality and safety of the care being rendered. At the same time, much remains to be done before Lewis Thomas's remarks lose their force.

As medical educators and thought leaders now routinely point out to budding clinicians,[11] patients frequently find their doctors' communication dissatisfying and/or fail to follow their doctors' instructions. Various studies have shown that between 10 and 70 percent of patients reject their doctors' advice about lifestyle changes and do not take their prescribed medications.

The modern history of communication between doctors and patients reveals significant flux. Many doctors used to think that it was bad for patients to know too much about their illnesses and treatments. Good patients did what they were told without question; troublesome ones who asked questions were undermining their confidence in their doctors[12] and thus damaging their care. Recent decades have brought a significant shift toward more liberal sharing of medical information with patients. Most people probably now understand that they own their medical information, because they must sign forms to allow it to be shared with their health insurance providers. It is always difficult to generalize about a complex situation in flux, because by the time a commentator makes an observation, it may no longer be current. However it is safe to say that we have a long way to go to implement effective, fail-safe methods of improving health information transfer across the populations of patients and potential patients.

The dynamics of communication between doctors and patients are receiving increasing attention from social scientists, medical educators, and others. But we are just beginning to explore the dynamics of developing of a trusting relationship between caregivers and patients who do not speak the same language or who come from different cultural backgrounds. Currently, it is beyond our capacity to deal with the subtleties and complexities of communication across multiracial and multilingual borders. The 2008 national elections augur a major cultural shift for our society, which seems to be awakening to the reality of our multiracial population and the particular challenges to our health and education systems in terms of equity in the way we distribute goods and services.

In a study of clinician-patient communication, J. K. Burgoon and colleagues[13] concluded that how the clinician communicates with the patient may be more important to patient satisfaction than the content of the communication itself. After interviewing 234 patients who had seen a primary care doctor within the previous six months, they found that greater patient satisfaction was associated with greater expressions of receptivity, immediacy, composure, similarity, and informality, as well as less dominance by the physician. In consultations characterized by these factors, patients trusted their physicians more, believed that the physicians were concerned about them, believed that they were well-informed, felt safe to disclose personal information, felt liked and accepted, and were more satisfied with the physicians' techniques. These factors also had a modest positive effect on patients' compliance with treatment plans and recommendations. One can easily see that non-English-speaking patients would be on the wrong end of the curve in terms of having trust and confidence in their physicians. This establishes an important agenda for physicians who care for patients with significant cultural and linguistic differences.

The Word: An Indispensable Diagnostic Tool

Not only does good communication between doctors and patients make patients more satisfied and happy, it also serves the critical function of giving clinicians the information they need to treat effectively. In Philip Tumulty's words:

> What the scalpel is to the surgeon, words are to the clinician. When he uses them effectively, his patients do well. If not, the results may well be disastrous . . . The wisdom of Thomas Aquinas, the logic of Newman, and the clinical genius of Osler will not be effective in making well a patient who does not understand why he is sick, or what he must do to get well.[14]

Likewise, Dana Atchley has written:

> Warmth and compassion break down the barriers of anxiety and fear that . . . can seriously inhibit the thoroughness of a diagnostic appraisal. If a patient feels that his problems are provocative, not only of scientific interest, but also of a deep concern over his happiness, he will be more open in discussing his life and his deeper feelings, and also more cooperative in accepting unpleasant diagnostic and therapeutic procedures. A good emotional rapport between the doctor and his patient improves his efficiency as a healer, and indeed, makes the whole process more pleasant.[15]

The patient-nurse interaction also elicits clinically relevant elements in the patient's history. Growing recognition of the importance of the nursing profession and its traditional emphasis on interpersonal and communication skills is expanding the role of the nurse on the health care team. One of many factors driving this development is the greater ethnic and cultural diversity of the nursing corps compared with the physician corps. The words of Tumulty and Atchley, written to describe caregivers and patients who speak the same language and share the same cultural background, are relevant to all clinical encounters. But achieving the desired trusting relationship with caregivers is much more complex for patients not fluent in English and for those from strikingly different cultural backgrounds. As the health care system encounters larger numbers of first-generation immigrants, our health teams must have access to people who can bridge the language and cultural divide, to help create a patient-oriented therapeutic care environment. Although medical school enrollments are becoming increasingly diverse, nurses will continue to be on the front lines of resolving this important issue.

George Engel, the professor of medicine and psychiatry at the University of Rochester renowned for his definition of the "biopsychosocial" paradigm, has described the patient interview as the most powerful, encompassing, sensitive, and versatile instrument in all of medicine.[16] The classical scientific paradigm that held sway from the time of Newton to that of Curie and Einstein portrayed what was being studied as external to and independent of the researcher, who discovered and objectively characterized its properties and behavior. Engel's biopsychosocial paradigm, in contrast, emerges from the idea that what is being studied is inseparable from the scientist, who devises mental constructs of his or her understanding of its properties and behavior. Engel's paradigm reflects the observation of Max Delbrück, cowinner of the 1969 Nobel Prize in Physiology or Medicine for his work on random mutation in bacterial resistance to viruses. What a scientist (or a physician) observes is not nature (or physiology) itself, but the interplay between nature and ourselves: science describes nature through to our way of questioning.[17]

In the late-1980s Jaroslav Pelikan, then provost of Yale University, similarly observed that reason is not the only way of knowing. He believed that university education should also respect and include other channels of insight and discovery, such as intuition and the emotions. In this regard we might well remember that Albert Einstein famously said, "Imagination is more important than knowledge," and that imagination is never strictly rational.

We live in what many observers call a postmodern, post-Enlightenment world. For some extreme relativists, this brings into question all the achievements of the Enlightenment and the evidence-based science that descends from it, including modern Western medicine. Certainly, if modern Western medicine is anything, it is a chief legacy of the Enlightenment and the crowning achievement of the modern Western industrialized, democratic society, which the Enlightenment did so much to shape.

Evidence, reason, and logic do not fly out the window when other ways of knowing come in, however. The evidence for the random processes of quantum physics has no less rigor than that for classical Newtonian physics, and biologists have mapped quantum processes at work in the everyday world of photosynthesis and enzyme reactions.

Our society will eventually find its way to a new synthesis of Enlightenment and post-Enlightenment, modern and postmodern thinking. In the meantime, today's health professionals can best help their patients to heal with words, the arts, and the senses, as well as the placebo effect (to which we'll turn in the next chapter) if they take an approach that is both open minded and evidence based regarding the diversity of ideas in our multicultural America.

Amy Chua's argument in *Day of Empire: How Hyperpowers Rise to Global Dominance—and Why They Fall*, that America's present and future strength lies in our diversity and tolerance, is one of several ideas,[18] along with those of Engel, Delbrück, and Pelikan, that shape my own approach. Another is historian Daniel Boorstin's description of America as "the Republic of Technology," in which we look to the next technological and scientific breakthroughs to keep us free from oppressions of all kinds.[19] I would also point to Robert Bellah's and colleagues' now classic book, *Habits of the Heart*, for its chronicling of the tension and interplay between American ideals of individualism and community[20]; Viktor Frankl's[21] and Dennis Ford's[22] separate delineations of the universal core and varied forms of all human beings' search for meaning in their lives; the philosopher Susan Neiman's trenchant observations, in *Moral Clarity: A Guide for Grown-Up Idealists*,[23] that the Enlightenment was intrinsically neither atheistic nor agnostic and that Kant's version of the golden rule, treat each person as an end and not a means, provides a strong, flexible principle for navigating the ambiguities and dilemmas of modern society; and the philosopher (and my old friend) John McDermott's view,[24] also espoused by Neiman, that the one nonrelative limit we all face is death and that we should do so with confidence in the unique value of each life and the communities we build together.

When any of us become convinced that our logic is unshakeable, we would do well to remember what neuroscience is demonstrating about the often irrational processes of the human mind. As Robert Burton reports in his book *On Being Certain: Believing You Are Right Even When You're Not*, certainty seems to be a feeling emerging from the amygdala, a more primitive part of the midbrain somewhat distant from the cerebral cortex, where logical reasoning apparently resides.[25] On the one hand, the feeling of certainty can be remarkably resistant to modification. When the cerebral cortex (reasoning) and the midbrain (feeling) are in nonnegotiable conflict, the certainty feeling triumphs. On the other hand, neuroscience experiments also show that the amygdala and cortex are inextricably connected and that their ties may be strengthened, indicating that good decision making involves collaboration between both parts of the brain.

To sum this up by paraphrasing a thought attributed to Einstein, which I believe applies strongly to our current health care system and its path to renewal: The intuitive mind is a sacred gift and the rational mind is a faithful servant, but our society honors the servant and neglects the gift.

Engel reminds me of that gift when he counsels that in an

encounter with a patient, the physician must operate concurrently in two modes—one observational, the other relational—each of which deals with different sorts of data. In the observational mode, the physician collects data observable through the senses or extensions thereof, like stethoscopes, blood pressure monitors, blood tests, X-rays, and MRI scans. In the relational mode, the physician collects data from the uniquely human realm of articulated language, symbols, thoughts, and feelings. Through this mode the physician may learn the nature and history of the patient's experiences and clarify what they mean to the patient and what they mean in other systems, be they psychological or social. The clarification of meaning achieved in the relational mode illuminates measurements taken in the observational mode to provide a clear and complete picture of the patient's symptoms.

Others agree that the clinician-patient interchange is the most potent tool for understanding a patient's illness and finding an appropriate treatment. Fletcher and Freeling, when they teach medical students how to talk and listen to patients, divide the consultation into two parts: the interview and the discussion (much along the lines of Engel's observational and relational modes). They emphasize the discussion as follows: "Doctors should not just tell patients about the diagnosis and proposals for management, but should first find out their views and discuss them in order to reach an agreed diagnosis and plan of action. Studies have shown that patients will be more likely to accept and carry out this plan if they have participated in its formulation."[26]

To those who argue that they don't have time for discussions, Fletcher and Freeling concede that good consultations may on average take more time than less good ones, but if this means they are more effective, they will save time in the long run. In my own experience as a patient with complex teams of nurses, doctors, and technicians, I have found that manifest interprofessional respect produces more effective, efficient, and frequent communication with the patient.

The success of that communication depends on sensitivity to the individual patient as well as on good teamwork between caregivers. During my years at the University of Washington, I was the house officer in charge of a young, diabetic, recently married woman. She had been referred by her general physician to Dr. Robert Williams, a deservedly world-famous endocrinologist who was the chairman of the department of internal medicine. The patient's main problem was weakness and faintness at night and early in the morning. Her equally young husband was appropriately attentive and anxious about his new wife's serious health issues. As we followed her over a four- or five-day period, adjusting her insulin dosages literally hour by hour on the basis of the frequent monitoring of her blood glucose levels, she proved to be very difficult to manage and her blood sugars in the morning were inexplicably dangerously low. I got to know the patient and her husband quite well during those days. I frequently checked the patient during the night along with careful twenty-four-hour monitoring by the nurses. In those days no visitors were allowed at night.

Very perplexed, Dr. Williams began to suspect that the patient was somehow receiving too much insulin during the nighttime hours. I reviewed in detail all the insulin orders and how the injections were given. When the patient was at X-ray, Dr. Williams took the patient's vial of injectable insulin from her bag of personal items and added a chemical tag that is excreted promptly in the urine. The next day's blood and urine tests solved the mystery. Her blood sugar levels showed a dangerous downturn and her urine contained the metabolic tag. Her husband could not have injected her with the extra insulin because he was not there during the time in question. If the nurses—they were all first-rate—had not done so, that left only the patient herself.

Discussing all this, Dr. Williams and I concluded that the newlywed patient was acting out of anxiety over securing her husband's loving concern and attachment. We also concluded that one of us would have to raise the issue when the husband arrived to visit his wife. Inasmuch as I had come to know the couple better and was much closer to them in age, I was left to conduct the meeting.

It seemed to me that a nonjudgmental approach was essential, and this triggered an idea that I acted on as follows. My first step was to share the good news that we had finally figured out the puzzle of the wife's early-morning low blood sugar problems. Explaining how we had ruled out any other possibility, I then said that nothing made sense, except that she was giving herself insulin during the night unconsciously, while she was asleep, and that we had proved this by inserting a chemical tag in her insulin. Adding that we believed she must be doing the same thing at home, but of course without knowing it, I told them we recommended that her husband take charge of the insulin at bedtime.

Judging by her immediate acceptance of this face-saving scenario, she very much liked the idea that she was a shot-giving sleepwalker (Dr. Williams also thought this a very neat explanation, when I shared it with him later). The couple and I then had a very healthy and positive discussion about their relief at knowing how to keep her blood sugar within bounds again.[27] Later, I sometimes wondered if the wife's behavior was only a matter of newlywed anxiety or if she kept trying to elicit extraordinary attention and care from her husband by other means, conscious or unconscious. After all, our silver-lining interpretation that she was doing it in her sleep might have been correct, but no less of an issue for that!

The Language of the Arts

Just as words can be used to understand others and to help them heal, so too can other forms of expression. The arts in particular provide a powerful medium for communicating thoughts and feelings. Art can also, like laughter and verbal assurance, make people feel good—inspired, relaxed, content. In short, art can be a healing force.

Attempts to understand or relate to artistic works of all sorts aid the clinician in developing a sensitivity to patients, thus enhancing the clinical ability to decipher both the verbal and nonverbal messages patients convey. Clinicians also find that regular exposure to the arts is not only pleasurable but helps them work out their capacity to handle their daily exposure to suffering and death. The arts, after all, are attempts at communication, usually of emotions and perceptions, precisely the skills area in which an increasing number of patients find many modern clinicians most deficient.[28] In a presentation at the University of Texas Health Sciences Center at Houston, artist and critic Jamake Highwater likened the suffering patient's need to connect with human understanding and compassion to that of the artist, who is like a blinking star in the sky trying to communicate with the other—enormously distant—blinking stars all around.

Psychotherapists frequently use art in therapy for young children, where verbal expression can be difficult. Asking children who suffer from cancer or other serious chronic diseases to draw themselves, their treatments, and their diseases leads to a better understanding of their feelings and thereby to the identification of emotional conflict that might be inhibiting their healing process.

Art can also be a source of positive feelings and hence a stimulant to our internal restorative mechanisms. We embrace the idea that the arts (finger paints, clay modeling, sand-castle building, ballet) may help young children learn, grow, and develop qualities like self-confidence and coordination. But our society is only just learning, partly in response to the aging of our population and the associated increase of chronic disease and debility, that the same activities benefit adult growth, happiness, and sometimes healing. Artists tell us that when they create something—a painting, a sculpture, a dance—they experience the very basic pleasures of bringing something to life and sharing a part of themselves with others. Herein art is a life force. It reminds the artist that he or she has the power to make things happen and is connected to others in our world. Such feelings of vitality, self-affirmation, and connectedness are precisely the sorts of feelings lost by people isolated by illness and the prospect or fear of death. Thus our aging population can find the arts increasingly useful in helping to cope with chronic illness and the evening of their lives.

The therapeutic value of art has gained increasing recognition over the past several decades. Programs to bring artists-in-residence to health care facilities have been created, and an area called "health care arts administration" has been developed, through which hospitals can become patrons of the arts for their therapeutic value.[29] Architects are designing newer hospitals to be airier and brighter, more spacious and colorful, with rooms that have windows and an outward orientation. Such hospitals succeed in feeling more like places for healing than places designed for isolation of the sick or dying. Patients are measurably better off if their rooms have windows.[30] As Guido Majno points out, it is difficult to rise above the daily routine when the eye cannot catch a glimpse of the sky.[31] The dramatic, long overdue switch to "building green" has been a great boon to creating a healthful environment for the provision of health care!

The Language of Music

The expressive and healing properties of the musical arts are perhaps the most widely recognized. Certain types of music are known to enhance healing and reduce pain. Music therapy is an established profession, the beginnings of which, according to music therapist John Beaulieu, can be traced back to the observations of a group of professional musicians who worked with returning World

War II veterans.[32] The musicians volunteered to perform in hospitals, with the intention of helping veterans pass their time in a pleasurable way. To their surprise, the musicians noticed that the patients who were exposed to music on a regular basis showed a marked increase in morale, as well as an improvement in socialization skills. Their depressions lifted faster as their suppressed emotions found a safe form of expression through music.

During the 1950s and 1960s, two professional associations dedicated to understanding the healing qualities of sound and music were formed.[33] These associations certify music therapists graduating from the seventy or so university training programs in music therapy. They also support research and work to increase public awareness of the benefits of music therapy. Today music therapists work in hospitals, clinics, and centers serving patients who are mentally challenged, physically handicapped, and learning disabled, in addition to those suffering from cancer, heart disease, and psychiatric conditions.

Musicians and orchestral conductors, who often perform into advanced age, frequently attribute their longevity to their love of music. Making music makes them feel "fully alive." Several have given testimony to having aching fingers grow more nimble and less painful as they play for the first time each day. Albert Schweitzer, who brought his grand piano with him to his medical clinic in equatorial Africa, said that playing the music of Johann Sebastian Bach freed him from the unremitting tensions of his days, restoring him to the ordered splendor he had always found in music. Music was his medicine and kept him working productively into old age as a physician. Claudius Conrad is a modern counterpart, a young neurosurgeon and highly accomplished pianist who works his best when listening to certain music. His area of research involves studying music's healing potential.

Three decades ago, I knew of no institutionally organized arts programs at academic health science and medical centers. When the University of Texas Health Science Center at Houston found the resources to start one in the 1980s, I believe that only Johns Hopkins Medical Center was similarly involved. The program brought the visual and performing arts to the Texas Medical Center in the form of periodic performances and lectures, which regularly attracted standing-room-only lunch-hour audiences. In a brown-bag lunch session held in one of the school's classrooms, the director of a local professional ballet troupe talked about ballet in preparation for the troupe's performance at the school the following day. I know nothing of ballet, but I learned more in that half hour about body language in particular and nonverbal communication in general, than I had in twenty years of clinical and teaching exposure. The troupe director demonstrated how her finishing gestures sent messages to the audience and explained how certain movements could elicit their response. Since her talk, I have become more adept at reading the body language of others. I have also gained a lasting awareness of the use of my own body language in one-on-one interactions and with groups, small or large. Over the past two decades, many more creative programs have been established within medical and health centers, hospitals and clinics across America.

In regard to the development of a healing relationship by using words or other forms of communication as therapy, I feel certain of only two things. First, it is a humbling subject that can engage any interested caregiver for a lifetime of learning and self-enhancement. Second, the ability to help others help themselves to reduce their suffering, or defeat their disease, has everything to do with building trust and confidence that the caregiver is accepting, nonjudgmental, and will stick with the patient until things are resolved. The caregiver, by word, body movement, or other sign of commitment, must demonstrate that she or he cares for the patient.

By the same token, the more the patient is engaged positively with others, the better. As a patient, I learned that I seemed to gain in my own health struggles when I focused on other people and their issues. I was reminded to try that approach when I read a comment the physician Lewis Thomas made from his deathbed. He said he believed that in general what human beings did best was to help others. Victor Frankl worked with debilitated people by encouraging them to find and express a personally transcendent goal. This philosophy has influenced countless para- and quadraplegic patients to find ways to encourage others in their time of trouble.

Thus, whatever interactions one enjoys with art, language, and communication can only enhance, directly or indirectly, one's capacity to be a consistently constructive, positive force in patients' attempts to regain health or minimize suffering. It all boils down to the so-called art of medicine. Communicating sincere interest in improving the patient's condition helps him or her feel more comfortable from the start. It is a healing act for both clinician and patient.

Good communication—the ability to make connections with a wide variety of people, many of whom speak different languages from ours—constitutes a critical challenge for science-based medicine, a challenge that must be shared among physicians, nurses, physician assistants, and other caregivers. The combination of good communication with almost magical technical interventions gives the modern-day physician the capacity to become the most potent and prolific healer of all time. The physician can't do it all, but if physicians don't work to create a collaborative, patient-sensitive listening environment for health care, the success of their therapeutic efforts will be diminished. And, without doubt, discerning, informed patients can vote with their feet if they perceive they are not a part of a healthful team. There are and will continue to be a growing number of health care providers capable of constructing a supportive, health-promoting patient care environment.

The therapeutic potential of words, art, and the senses ultimately rests on the body's capacity for self-healing. Let's look at how the placebo effect may also trigger this capacity.

Chapter 3

Self-Healing, Our Internal Pharmacy, and the Placebo Effect

In the midnineteenth century, Oliver Wendell Holmes said that if all the medicines in the world were thrown into the sea, it would on balance be bad for the fish and good for the people. A little later, a French physician provided a more ironic perspective on the same general issue by declaring that clinicians should use all newly available treatments as widely and as often as possible, before they became ineffective. In the midtwentieth century, L. J. Henderson, the famed Harvard biochemist, may have been satirizing his own need for improbable precision by saying, "Somewhere between 1910 and 1912 in this country, a random patient, with a random disease, consulting a doctor chosen at random, had for the first time in the history of mankind a better than fifty-fifty chance of profiting from the encounter."[1] Clearly, medicine has had its trials as well as its triumphs.

Given the historical ineffectiveness—and in some cases downright danger—of medical treatments and procedures, what accounts for the perceived success of medicine and high status of physicians throughout the centuries? A major part of the answer may be found in a review of placebos.

I believe the often heated discussion about placebos in medicine wastes a good deal of energy because of a failure to agree on the definition of "placebo" and "placebo effect." A. K. Shapiro defines a placebo as follows:

> Any therapeutic procedure (or that component of any procedure) which is given deliberately to have an effect, or unknowingly has an effect on a patient, symptom, syndrome, or disease, but which is objectively without specific activity for the condition being treated. The therapeutic procedure may be given with or without conscious knowledge that the procedure is a placebo, may be an active (non-inert) or non-active (inert) procedure, and includes therefore all medical procedures no matter how specific.[2]

The "placebo effect" simply refers to the outcome – favorable or unfavorable – that a placebo, as defined by Shapiro, produces in the person who receives it.

The placebo effect may be subjective or may have objective physiologic manifestations.[3, 4, 5] These manifestations can include an increase in endorphins, which reduces pain, as well as increases in the vitality and effectiveness of the immune system's T-cells or macrophages, which can directly ameliorate and sometimes cure disease. Researchers typically describe the placebo effect as revolving around three factors: the beliefs and expectations of the patient, the beliefs and expectations of the physician, and the nature and quality of the patient-physician relationship.[6, 7, 8] I would expand the third factor to include the nature and quality of the patient-clinician relationship and the caregiving environment. This takes account of dentists, nurses, physician associates, psychologists, physical therapists, and others on the clinical team as well as physical elements in the caregiving environment.

A review by Turner and colleagues of the literature on placebos supports the potential value of expanded research on the placebo effect. They found that placebo response rates vary considerably and are often much higher than the frequently cited 30 to 40 percent. They point out that placebos tend to have time-effect curves, with peak, cumulative, and carryover effects resembling those of active medications. They also concluded that individuals tend to be inconsistent in their placebo responses and that no "placebo-responder" personality has been identified.[9] Labeling a patient who has responded positively to a placebo a "placebo-responder" falsely implies a psychological predisposition for which there is no evidence.

Given individuals' inconsistent placebo responses, we might well ask whether a change of physician plays a role. Perhaps we should be identifying some physicians as "placebo response elicitors." To my knowledge, no one has studied individual clinicians' ability to elicit beneficial placebo responses from their patients, although much has been written on the value of trust in establishing a therapeutic relationship.

The essential mechanism of the placebo effect resides in the intersection of belief with pathophysiologic and molecular biologic processes. In the simplest form of placebo, a clinician gives a patient an inactive pill, or one not known to affect the patient's particular symptoms (or at least some of them); the patient takes the pill hoping or believing that it will relieve symptoms, and it does. Not limited to treatment in the form of pills, the placebo effect can occur after any treatment, even surgery, which the patient and the physician believe is effective. Three sets of studies from the literature on placebos and the placebo effect illuminate the fascinating and important link between psychological and physiological processes.

The first set of studies addresses "bone pointing," a phenomenon that baffled me when I encountered it during my service as a chief medical resident. A seventy-eight-year-old grandmother entered the hospital with a history and physical, and a few laboratory findings suggesting she had cancer. Although obviously worried about this possible diagnosis, she was a very cheerful, alert lady, and everyone involved in her care loved her.

After her initial workup and a battery of tests, she remained in the hospital awaiting the biopsy results, which we told her would be available in a few days. Meanwhile, we all saw her every day and she remained in good spirits. On the third day, however, the house staff told her the biopsy results would be three days late. While we waited for the report to come, she became insane. She made no sense, didn't recognize any of her caregivers or family, appeared both anxious and depressed, and wouldn't eat. None of us knew what to do.

A psychiatrist saw her but was unable to offer a remedy. One day later, the pathology report on her biopsy came back and was, if anything, worse than we all feared. After a brief discussion about whether to tell her the results, since she didn't seem to understand anything, the intern went in, sat at her bedside, and said the test showed she had a bad cancer and there was no treatment any of our specialists could recommend. On hearing this news, she snapped out of her mental confusion and into her old organizing self, getting the family and herself ready for her death. She called her relatives to her bedside and together they made plans for the next steps in her life and theirs.

Following her discharge the next day, my colleagues and I asked the psychiatrist if he could diagnose this strange episode. His explanation made us aware of a communication fault that had inflicted three days of mental and emotional suffering on the patient. In the psychiatrist's analysis, when we told our cheerful, alert patient that the biopsy report would not be coming for another three days, she lost faith that she was in trustworthy hands. She assumed we were withholding the results and abandoning her to die.

The psychiatrist then described how in some tribal cultures the act of a medicine man or woman pointing a bone at and cursing someone could so convince the person of his or her imminent death that death did indeed occur in a matter of days or weeks. The psychiatrist also related the practice of tree shaking. In some nomadic cultures, people above a certain age or below a certain obvious standard of strength had to try to climb a tree and stay in it while young men shook it back and forth. When the community moved on, whoever could not climb the tree or had fallen out of it was left behind to die.

Fearing she had an incurable condition, but denied the expected confirmation of this fact, our patient felt as she might have had we subjected her to bone pointing or tree shaking. Telling her the biopsy result restored her sense that we took her seriously and wanted to do all we could for her. In her eyes, it returned her to normal membership in society and enabled her to make good use of the time she had left.

In a classic 1942 article, the great physiologist Walter B. Cannon memorably described rapid deaths induced by bone pointing in previously healthy individuals.[10] Western medicine seemed powerless to alter the downhill course of the syndrome or identify a disease that explained its symptoms and signs. One case involved a perfectly healthy young man who began to die when he became convinced that, two years previously, he had been tricked into eating a food forbidden by a lethal curse. The man traced a rapid path downward, neither eating nor speaking. His Western friends tried everything to reverse the trend, but their efforts were of no avail. Finally, they found the man's tribal medicine man and bribed him to tell their friend that the gods had revoked the prohibition on the food he had eaten and that the spell was removed. Near death by all physiologic measures, the young man immediately brightened up, began to eat and talk, and soon recovered completely. Cannon took a particular interest in this case because the subject in question was one of his own laboratory technicians.

Researchers have observed such self-directed deaths in modern cultures as well. For example, clinicians know that long-married people often die shortly after their spouses do. Engel studied rapid death

during times of psychological stress,[11] and Milton studied self-willed
death in patients with melanoma.[12]

Another set of relevant studies, conducted by Stewart Wolf and
his colleagues, focuses on the placebo effect in gastrointestinal physiology and pharmacology. In one study, Wolf used pressure-record-
ing devices to study gastric contraction patterns in several human
subjects at rest, during digestion, and during times of nausea and
vomiting. In subjects stricken with nausea and vomiting, he was able
to show that the administration of ipecac, a medicine that induces
vomiting, had different effects based upon the information given to
the subjects. When subjects were openly given ipecac and informed
that it induced vomiting, they vomited as expected. When the subjects
were given ipecac but told that it was "an unnamed agent" that relieved nausea and prevented vomiting, their symptoms abated. Wolf
concluded:

> Placebo effects which modify the pharmacologic action of
> drugs or endow inert agents with potency are not imaginary,
> but may be associated with measurable changes at the end
> organs. These effects are at times more potent than the phar-
> macologic action customarily attributed to the agent. Thus
> the familiar difficulty of evaluating in patients new thera-
> peutic agents stems not only from inadequately curbed en-
> thusiasm of the investigator, but also from the actual
> physiologic effects of their 'placebo' action.[13]

In a subsequent investigation, Wolf and Pinsky studied thirty-one
patients with a variety of chronic disorders, all with a heavy overlay of
symptoms related to anxiety and tension. Each patient alternately
received a placebo and the test agent, which was purported to reduce
anxiety and tension, in a manner blind to both patient and physician.
The researchers found that regardless of whether the treatment was the

test agent or the placebo, about 15 percent of the patients got better, 70–75 percent stayed the same, and 10–12 percent got worse after each treatment.

Many of the subjects in the study reported vague and minor side effects; three had major reactions. One had overwhelming weakness, palpitation, and nausea within fifteen minutes of medication and another suffered several symptoms, including watery diarrhea within ten minutes, regardless of whether they had been given the test agent or the placebo. A third patient developed a diffuse, itchy rash after ten days of medication. When the medication was stopped, the rash disappeared, but the patient refused to participate further, even though the rash had occurred as a result of the placebo administration.[14] These findings point to the power of the mind to affect real and sometimes dramatic physical symptoms.

A third set of studies on the relationship between psychology and physiology is summarized in a 1989 research briefing, *Behavioral Influences on the Endocrine and Immune Systems*, published by the Institute of Medicine of the National Academy of Sciences. Among other substantial scientific evidence that behavior influences the immune system both directly and through the endocrine system, the briefing relates that bereaved men experience decreased immune function immediately following the death of their wives.[15] Kiecolt-Glaser and Glaser uncovered similar relationships between stressful life events and changes in the strength of the immune system.[16] Pert et al. build a case for the existence of a communications network of chemical interactions mediated by neuropeptides and their receptors, which join endocrine glands, the brain, and the immune system in what amounts to the biochemical substrate of emotion.[17]

Developments in modern neurochemistry, neuroendocrinology, and neuropsychoimmunology allow us to envision at a molecular level how emotions and beliefs can influence everything from white blood cell function to cardiovascular events to a host of other signs and symptoms. Dr. Elizabeth Sternberg of the National Institutes of Health has done an interesting neurosciences review in her recently published book, *Healing Spaces*, which has opened my eyes to how the visual pathways and connections can work to our advantage in healing. Images formed on the retina are transmitted to the visual cortex at the back of the brain. Research referred to by Dr. Sternberg has shown that there is a switch in the visual cortex sending different kinds of images to different parts of the cerebral cortex for storage. For example, images of human faces are known to be sent from their first stop in the visual cortex to a particular area in the brain for storage and easy recognition later if one sees that face or a photograph of that face. When the eye takes in a scene in the countryside or at a lake or mountain that is pleasurable, like those printed on the Bedscapes drapes I described in the previous chapter, that image rides along the same optic nerve from the retina to the visual cortex, where it is sent on via a different neuronal path toward a cerebral site different from where individual faces are stored. This storehouse, when activated, rings up high on the pleasantness meter as experienced by the host individual.

Sternberg reports that the neuron leading to this pleasurable scene recollection center is lined with endorphin granules that are released as the message runs closer to the storage site. Apparently, the closer the neuron is to the cortical storage center, the more packed endorphins there are, ready for release by the neuron.[18] These studies, along with similar findings on auditory messages such as music, position the art of medicine as an emerging science through which the adept practitioner encourages the patient's own internal pharmacy to dispense agents in therapeutic combinations and amounts at just the right time.

The patient's faith in the doctor, not the pill, seems to be the most powerful force operating in the placebo effect. Physician and popular writer about the mind-body connection Bernie Siegel describes the role of the faith healer in primitive medicine and the somewhat analogous role of the modern Western physician as a source of inspiration for self-healing. He writes:

> Nearly all so-called primitive medicines use the placebo factor via rituals that foster assurance in the healing force, whether it is defined as an external god or an internal energy. Faith healing relies on the patient's belief in a higher power and the healer's ability to act as a channel to it. Sometimes a mere artifact or saint's relic is conduit enough. For a believer a bottle labeled as Lourdes holy water has healing properties even if there's only tap water in it ... This is why it's so important that a physician have ... the ability to project confidence. A patient's hope and trust lead to a "letting go" that counteracts stress and is often the key to getting well.[19]

Many experienced clinicians and patients alike agree that a trusting relationship is more important, in the long run, than any medicine or procedure. But a patient's faith in the doctor can also produce negative effects, as for example when physicians yield to the patient's desire to know how much longer they can expect to live. In many cases, patients die right on schedule, as if they were attempting to validate their perception of the doctor's assessment or alternatively as if the bone had been figuratively pointed at them. For this reason, most physicians believe it is generally better not to be too precise about a possible timetable for death.

Why then, when observations like these have been repeatedly made, and when so many studies on the placebo effect indicate that it leads to a 30 to 40 percent (some claim 50 to 60 percent) improvement rate in almost any symptom, has this important tool been ignored or denigrated for so long? We probably cannot overestimate the influence of the Hippocratic tradition on physicians' image of themselves and their profession as acting solely upon a rational understanding of historical data and physical facts.[20]

Since the Second World War, what we may properly call the biomolecular revolution has swept forward with dramatic results, touching virtually all our lives. One gene, one protein, one disease, one precise cure! These words describe the central concept of reductionist biomedicine. This paradigm has produced increasingly effective tools, which have which have rendered such dramatic results that the focus of our attention has become the tools and not the healer or the healed. The genome project is perhaps the ultimate expression of the reductionist theory. Although the genome project has already added immensely to our knowledge and will surely prove well worth the effort expended on it, evidence increasingly indicates that most diseases are not caused by single genes. Multiple genetic factors are probably more often at work, along with organismal and environmental factors.

Generations of doctors have now been trained under the pervasive influence of the tremendous successes of the biomedical revolution, which has seemed to hold out the promise of perpetual improvement. In that context, physicians have come to regard placebos and the placebo effect in a cavalier manner, if not with outright disdain. Many mature physicians have grown up considering that a patient cured by a placebo is something less than a real patient, whose ailment demands the proper chemotherapeutic agent or surgical intervention, and that a doctor whose work is done through the placebo is something less than a real doctor. Early in my clinical career, I thought this way, as did many of my peers and colleagues.

Americans have a strong cultural belief in advanced technology. We count on our capacity to control or intervene effectively in nature. Yet most accepted, standard medical practice consists of interventions that have not been statistically proven to be effective using randomized placebo-controlled trials.

Recent exploration of the placebo effect has probably had a

positive impact on patients' health by placing renewed emphasis on the quality of the clinician-patient relationship. Physician Howard Spiro describes this impact:

> [W]e physicians live in two worlds: the world of science, which provides us with our ideals and with real advances against disease, and the world of people, persons with instincts, with pain, suffering, hope, and joy. We have a hard time separating out what we learn in science from what we need to know in practice to deal with people. The placebo reminds us to focus on the interface between those two worlds ... What the placebo effect does is to act as a symbol of a connection—tangible evidence that some person cares and will try to do something.[21]

Spiro, like Arthur Kleinman and others, points to the important differences between disease and illness. The placebo does not treat the disease on a molecular level; rather, it treats the associated illness as it affects a particular patient.

A placebo effect may reduce the pain and suffering associated with a disease. For example, although the curative treatment for acute bacterial pneumonia will be a specific antibiotic, the symptoms and the overall impact of the disease can vary tremendously from patient to patient. Changes in the clinical impact of the illness can come not only from the antibiotic, but from other medical and therapeutic interventions utilized, including the placebo effect.

In my years of clinical practice, my working rule of thumb was that giving a placebo in a randomized clinical trial might have a positive effect in 40 percent of cases. However, if the patient believed the treatment would help, the positive responses would rise to 60–65 percent. If both the patient and the physician believed in the treatment's effectiveness, the positive responses would be in the 80–90 percent range.

A dramatic example of this phenomenon played itself out in the 1950s and 1960s in studies of the ligation of the internal mammary artery, in order to redirect blood into the nearby coronary arteries. Experiments in dogs showed that blood flow through the coronary arteries significantly increased when surgery closed off the nearby internal mammary artery.

On the basis of these animal studies, one of America's leading surgeons began to treat a series of patients suffering from serious, often debilitating angina pectoris with internal mammary artery ligation. This achieved success wonderful results at first, with people in 90 percent of cases becoming symptom free and returning to work. As other doctors picked up on this approach, their success rates were also high, but in some instances only in the 60–65 percent range.

At this point, a team of my teachers and eventual colleagues at the University of Washington in Seattle, led by cardiologist Len Cobb and thoracic surgeons David Dillard and K. Alvin Merendino, courageously undertook a randomized trial comparing internal mammary ligation and a sham operation. The sham operation proceeded to the point of placing the ligature around the internal mammary artery. But instead of tightening and tying a knot in the ligature, thus restricting blood flow into the artery as in the real operation, the surgeons removed the ligature and sewed the patient back up, leaving blood flow in the internal mammary artery unrestricted. In this trial, the positive clinical response rate, as determined by decreased angina, increased exercise tolerance, return to work, and sense of well-being, was the same in both the operated and sham-operated groups of patients, without around 45 percent of the patients in each group showing improvement.

Internal mammary ligation was not used after the randomized trial and never became a regular treatment option. When some of the trial patients who received the sham operation and experienced clinical improvement as a result were informed that their surgery had not included actual internal mammary ligation, they seemed unfazed by the news. They still felt cured and were very glad of the surgery they did have. A more recent example on a less dramatic scale is described in a randomized study report of the effectiveness of arthroscopic surgery in treating osteoarthritis of the knee, which concludes that surgery was no more effective than a sham operation.[22]

A recent survey of internists and rheumatologists caring for chronically ill patients has shown that a majority of them prescribe medicines they think are unlikely to do any good except through the placebo effect.[23] Because there is no indication they will stop such treatment, we can expect to have some lively discussions on the ethics of placebo administration. I believe the stopping of the internal mammary procedure was correct and ethically justified and that providing hope and sometimes a symptomatic improvement with a relatively safe and inexpensive pill will generally be acceptable to patients and doctors alike.

The issue of developing a proper therapeutic doctor-patient relationship leads us to the phenomenon of transference. William Zinn describes transference phenomena in the physician-patient relationship and its power to affect health as follows:

> Transference is a process in which individuals displace patterns of behavior that originate through interaction with significant figures in childhood onto other persons in their current lives. It is a powerful determinant of patient behavior in medical encounters. Transference can affect the kind of physician-patient relationship a patient seeks and his or her response to interventions prescribed by physicians . . . Transference issues can also affect level of somatization and patient adherence to medical regimens.[24]

Thus experienced clinicians know to remain keenly sensitive not only to their own role in a transference process with another person but also to the variations that different patients bring to such encounters. One of the trickiest and subtlest of the various arts of medicine for clinicians is the ongoing challenge of handling these relationships.

Some have expressed concern about complications that the use of placebos may introduce into the clinician-patient relationship. The ethicist Sissela Bok argues categorically against giving patients sugar pills or other inert substances while claiming they are true medicines. Bok includes this in a broader argument that lying is always immoral in her book *Lying: Moral Choice in Public and Private Life.*

If our understanding of the placebo effect is broadened, however, to take into account that it can occur with any therapeutic intervention—involving either inert or active substances—then giving the medicine in the hope that it will improve the patient's condition does not constitute a lie and seems to me clearly acceptable and ethically justifiable. Surely the end, the patient's improved health, justifies the means, an inert substance, when so much evidence shows that it can be as truly medicinal as an active one. Much depends on how the clinician presents the medicine to the patient. Saying that it has proven helpful to others with the same problems and may well help the patient, too, is quite different from guaranteeing its efficacy. Experienced clinicians generally avoid such guarantees in any event, because no medicine works the same for every patient.

The 2008 Declaration of Helsinki generally limits the ethical use of placebos as the measure of comparison for the effectiveness of new drugs, whereas the U. S. Food and Drug Administration (FDA) endorses the International Conference of Harmonization's Good Clinical Practices, which allow for placebo-based trials. Spiro describes some of the practical hazards of placebo use by physicians, one of the most serious being that clinicians may delude themselves into thinking that a patient has no significant disease because a placebo has successfully relieved pain or other symptoms.[25] Worse yet, the clinician may also conclude that a placebo response indicates that the original complaint was feigned. In either case, successful placebo treatment could engender false security or complacency in future instances of disease in a particular patient.

In my experience as a caregiver and a patient, there has never been a need to use an inert sugar pill as a placebo. Even in the darkest times, there is always something to give, perhaps even an unexpected cure, that offers hope for relief of pain or other troublesome symptoms until the point is reached when there is nothing to do but provide comfort. When that point is reached, the doctor must say so and act accordingly.

Although it is always a surprise, health professionals must bear in mind that even some far advanced cancers will regress and so-called spontaneous remissions or cures occur, which confounds the placebo phenomenon even further. Hope is the counterpoint to our death, and caregivers must assist patients as they seek to adjust their realistic hopes against the inevitability of death. It is important to note that our multicultural and minority patient populations present challenges to our system at the end of life. In an optimal situation, caregivers will be able to respond to the chronically ill and elderly in a culturally sensitive way so that no one needs to die alone and abandoned. This underscores the need to diversify the health professional workforce as quickly as we are able.

In summary, we seem to have come full circle. Medical science has generated spectacular new technologies, many of which are commonly accepted despite being largely unproven in terms of effectiveness, especially in comparison to the placebo effect. These technologies may command the fervent belief of physicians and the public, and future anthropologists may well conclude that our current high-tech, highly interventionist, specialty oriented American health care system is actually a highly mechanized placebo. I personally don't believe in such a conclusion, because so much of what we do actually works and because our capacity to make effectiveness determinations is growing. However, we must recognize and sustain the placebo effect and not squander the public trust, thus reducing the placebo effect's built-in success rate. Our goal is patient healing, not placebo-free healing. It is more important to learn all we can as quickly as we can about the mind-body relationship. If we can understand how individuals' beliefs can enable them—not the doctor—to cure themselves, then we will have hit on real healing, and that could enable us to teach others how to heal themselves.

As I have already noted, research on the placebo effect has focused more upon patient susceptibility and the nature of the intervention than upon the skill of caregivers in developing a relationship of trust with patients, which is essential to all healing. Recent and laudatory changes in medical school education focus on teaching this skill. It has long been a core objective in nursing education, and it must become an operative core in developing the spirit of the evolving health care team. Focusing almost solely upon the education of the physician, a trap into which I have frequently fallen in the past, fails to address the major issues surrounding our population's cultural diversity. Not only is a largely Caucasian medical, dental, and nursing workforce confronted by the cultural differences inherent in America's black, Latino, and Asian minorities, but we currently have one immigrant for every eight native-born Americans, the highest percentage since the 1920s. As a patient, I know I want every treatment to work and care not whether it is the drug's, my caregivers', or my own molecules that do most in getting the therapeutic goal accomplished. Furthermore, the more diverse my team of caregivers is, the better I like it, in part because I know that in relatively short order there will be no ethnic majority group in America. Everyone will belong to one minority or another.

America is known for its pragmatism in the overall thrust to improve our lives. It may be that we should worry less about whether a medication is or is not a placebo and focus instead on efforts to release and enhance patients' intrinsic healing capacities.

Chapter 4

Understanding Suffering

Illness is the night-side of life, a more onerous citizenship. Everyone who is born holds dual citizenship, in the kingdom of the well and in the kingdom of the sick. Although we all prefer to use only the good passport, sooner or later each of us is obliged, at least for a spell, to identify ourselves as citizens of that other place.

Susan Sontag, *Illness as Metaphor*

We spend much of our lives trying to avoid suffering, but sooner or later it finds us all. Since it is part of the human condition to suffer, we all ought to be equally qualified to consider suffering, and as a society we should collectively expend more of an effort to come to grips with it emotionally and intellectually. Health professionals, especially doctors and nurses, have extensive experience with the suffering of "patients," a word that also connotes suffering or endurance. Although there are gradations one can use to describe the levels and characteristics of pain—and pain is a form of suffering—suffering itself is very much a qualitative and subjective thing. This becomes easy for caregivers to overlook, especially if they feel helpless or incompetent to deal with it. From my earliest days as a hospital-based intern in internal medicine, I came to assume that just going into the hospital as a patient was a potentially life-threatening event. Thus I tried from the outset to identify patients' fears about being in the hospital setting. I firmly believe that such an approach helped reduce the collateral suffering around the hospital experience.

Another aspect of suffering is its impact on the rest of a person's life. After I had a bout with lymphoma, prospective employers and headhunters suddenly stopped calling me. Because I was sixty-one at the time and only wanted to complete my tenure at the Association of Academic Health Centers, this really didn't register with me until a woman academic leader asked whether anyone had solicited my interest in a new position since it became known I'd had cancer. A similar diagnosis at an earlier age had put the brakes on her career options, a situation she reversed only with great difficulty.

That was when I tuned in to the concern of patients of every age about how their medical experiences would affect their personal and professional lives. Such thoughts should naturally turn us toward new ties or the further development of existing ones. Along these lines, Richard Cohen has profiled several patients with chronic incurable and progressive diseases, who continue to develop new activities and relationships. Their example shows how we can help patients address this issue by providing a sympathetic ear and advice about a subject many people avoid.

When I was resting alone at home on the days after my cyclical chemotherapy for lymphoma, it shocked me that I suddenly started to cry several times. Feelings of helplessness, desolation, and fear bubbled up to the surface without warning. It brought home the realization that this might truly be the beginning of the end before I was fully prepared to deal with it. It encouraged me to remember the elderly lady, mentioned in the last chapter's discussion of bone pointing, who maintained her ability to connect with the world, and to take leave of it on her terms, so long as she felt that her caregivers took her seriously and spoke to her honestly. I knew that my caregivers, as well as my family and friends, treated me that way and would be there for me, no matter what happened.

This personal experience comes to mind when I consider physician Eric Cassel's description of suffering as a state of distress induced by the loss or threatened loss of control or meaning in one's life, or by the perceived disintegration of one's persona. Suffering, he relates, is a feeling that goes beyond and is distinct from pain. Two persons may be exposed to the same pain but suffer to different degrees. Suffering may also occur in the absence of pain, as in the anticipation of future pain. Cassel emphasizes the social and psychological foundations of suffering when he writes, "Suffering is a consequence of personhood—bodies do not suffer, persons do."[1]

Many authors have noted the linkage of suffering with a fear of death, separation, or isolation.[2, 3] Fortunato underscores the idea of the sufferer being excluded or feeling isolated from society in his book on the spiritual dilemma that the AIDS epidemic has forced upon society. He describes how an individual's suffering is dramatically heightened when social support systems seem to wither away as death becomes inevitable.[4] Vieth also deals with these ideas in terms of their theological implications,[5] which are included in our discussion because a large part of our society is influenced by theological considerations.

Margaret Mead, the iconic anthropologist, contended that all suffering citizens must be included in the fabric of society, to reduce their suffering as well as to increase the strength of society.[6] Implicit in this argument is the assumption that a strong society takes care of its weakest members. As poet William Blake wrote two centuries ago, "A dog starv'd at his master's gate / Predicts the ruin of the state."

Loss of self-respect greatly magnifies suffering, suggests Howard

Brody in his book *Stories of Illness*.[7] Conversely, helping patients maintain their self-respect can reduce their suffering.

American historian and Harvard University president Drew Gilpin Faust has published a widely acclaimed history of death and dying in the Civil War. She shows that this intense societal experience with suffering, death, and dying continues to exert profound influences upon America.[8] Thinking of the horribly painful deaths endured by so many at that time makes me appreciate the core of wisdom expressed by the thinkers and writers I have mentioned, but it also tells me that the discussion of suffering must include the problem of pain. We have made amazing strides in pain treatment over the last two centuries and our patients should have full advantage of them. A definitive analysis of our society's relationship to suffering must be left to scholars with a wider range than I can offer. I hope this chapter's observations on Americans' ideas about suffering in our increasingly diverse society may be useful and provocative. Exploring some of the ways in which our society is insensitive to suffering, may be promoting suffering, or is failing to ameliorate suffering may help us to take steps to improve our cultural environment.

Individualism and Self-Determination

Life, liberty, the pursuit of happiness, individuality, self-sufficiency: these are among the most fundamental of American values. Most people who voluntarily came to America left their own countries because they were poor, persecuted, desperately unhappy with their governments, or extremely ambitious. Those who were dragged here in chains or whose native lands were taken from them by the new arrivals could not be expected to look with favor upon their situation. Thus we are a nation famous for our inherent historical distrust in the collectivity, especially as it is reflected in the federal government.

America is renowned for upward mobility, although the possibilities for that have decreased of late, and the current recession has made us less optimistic about the future in general. Yet we have historically seen our standard of living go up, first through westward expansion to our frontiers and then through the Industrial Revolution and into the postindustrial era, and we continue to be a hopeful society. Our belief in self-reliant individualism can spawn the perception that people in unfortunate circumstances brought them upon themselves, are too lazy to change their situation, or are the inevitable losers in a survival-of-the-fittest economy. But it also makes us believe that everyone should have as many years as possible to enjoy life, liberty, and the pursuit of happiness, as enshrined in the Declaration of Independence. In that context, focusing on suffering could almost be considered unpatriotic. Why dwell on suffering? Better to forestall, delay, or deny its existence as long as possible.

Our commitment to the individual is reflected in our health care system and expenditures as well. It is seen most clearly in our love for dramatic innovations aimed at the saving of even one life or reducing the daily suffering of even one person, as exemplified in the recent attention to face transplantation. Our nation is capable of spending millions of dollars and riveting national attention for weeks on efforts to recover a child who has fallen into a well or a person lost at sea or in the mountains. To save a single premature infant, we routinely spend enough to prevent a large number of premature births in disadvantaged population groups. Of course, we can spend at both ends of the care spectrum, but we worry more about spending than about equal access to basic care for every American. We still haven't demonstrated that we believe health care is fundamentally a moral issue and only secondarily an economic consideration.

Arthur Kleinman, in his insightful book *The Illness Narratives*, expresses a different perspective: "Perhaps North American culture's ideology of personal freedom and the pursuit of happiness has come to mean, for many, guaranteed freedom from the suffering of pain. This meaning clashes strikingly with the expectation in much of the non-industrialized world that pain is an expected component of living and must be endured in silence."[9]

Ben Franklin's *Poor Richard's Almanac* epitomized Americans' reverence for individualism. "God helps those who help themselves," he wrote. Americans have taken these words to heart. When the aristocratic French historian and politician Alexis de Tocqueville described his visit to the young American republic in his 1835 book *Democracy in America*, he worried about the implications for Americans of their rampant individualism. He saw a growing number of Americans who believed they could handle the world with their family and their gun and their good sense and industry; they had no need for community. In *Habits of the Heart*, Robert Bellah and colleagues echo de Tocqueville, remarking that "Western culture for these last centuries . . . has obscured the more basic truth that we live in a sea of others without whom existence is literally unthinkable."[10]

Efficiency

Organization, linear behavior, and efficiency are integral features of the American work ethic and American success in the modern era. We work hard, move a lot, and sacrifice much in the name of efficiency, greater productivity, and greater profits. When a family member dies, we are supposed to get over it after a day or two and return to work with little or no emotion and a minimum of inconvenience for our coworkers. Grieving is not productive. Moreover, it disrupts the equilibrium of a finely tuned corporate or business organizational system. In this context, prolonged suffering seems to intrude on others and suggest that disappearing may be the most considerate thing for a suffering person can do for friends and colleagues.

Fighting Spirit

Americans admire fighters and those who portray fighters: John Wayne, Clint Eastwood, Muhammad Ali, Jackie Robinson, Martina Navratilova, Rambo, and even some famous politicians like Edward Kennedy. We celebrate our friends, relatives, ancestors, and heroes and heroines who fought their way out of poverty, ignorance, and hardship to attain better lives. Many of us have a sense that God not only helps those who help themselves, but that God loves a fighter! People who do not fight their diseases, we may believe at some level, are losers. Even children with cancer are taught to visualize their healthy cells destroying their cancer cells, and their success at visualizing this depends on their getting mad at the cancer cells. In addition, since a good fighter should not be afraid, we tend to avoid the difficult issues posed by suffering and the fear of personal dissolution and instead focus on bravery. Further, and perhaps most destructive, when suffering cannot be avoided and death seems inevitable, the sufferer may tend to feel like a failure for being unable to ward off the evil.

Loss of Community

Much damage has been done in recent decades to our ties to the social institutions—churches, clubs, home towns, communities, and families—that provided structure and support in the past. Some say we are even bowling alone these days! In place of community, our culture emphasizes personal privacy and individual rights and freedoms. In guarding our individuality, we pay less attention to the beliefs and values we share.

If suffering is a sort of separation that may be relieved by reincorporation into the group, the disintegration of social ties that link individuals to communities can only tend to make our culture increasingly unresponsive and insensitive to suffering in general. Suffering gets interpreted as an individual problem, leading to an isolation that ultimately exacerbates suffering. This seclusion, notes Eric Cassel, can further disrupt those aspects of personhood that require social contact: "Otherness is implied by self and many by one."[11] As recognized by proponents of twelve-step and other group-centered therapeutic approaches used in mental health settings, sharing fears, feelings, and experiences can be a powerful tool for combating suffering.

Belief That Suffering Is Punishment

Many Americans believe at some level that suffering is just punishment for sin and that the sufferer deserves to be shunned and lose dignity before the rest of society. Religious belief systems can be part of this reaction to suffering; the issues of suffering and pain are often entwined with the concept of evil in some religious explanations of the nature and intentions of God. Some religions teach that we deserve our suffering—that we suffer for original sin as well as for our individual transgressions. Many religions also suggest that the evil or sin that precipitated the suffering is contagious. These beliefs have important implications for the sufferer. Elizabeth Heitman notes that when "suffering is interpreted as punishment, a necessary lesson, or an inevitable consequence of nature," its association with evil may prompt others to reject the sufferer as contaminated and "the intervention of outsiders may be rejected as interference with the mechanism of cosmic justice."[12] This serves to further isolate the sufferer, who, as we have already seen, has plenty of other reasons to feel separated.

Patients whose afflictions are the result of socially unacceptable practices, such as substance abuse, sexual promiscuity, and, perhaps increasingly, smoking, may be more likely than other patients to have their suffering disregarded by people in a position to help, or ameliorate their discomfort. This may be especially true in settings where other suffering patients need attention. There is no doubt that it is far easier for a caregiver to feel empathy for the patient whose illness is unavoidable than for the patient who is returning for the fourth or fifth time with a behaviorally induced disorder. But caregivers need to remind themselves that much of what we consider at a surface level to be behaviorally associated, may be rooted in metabolic disorders beyond conscious control and free will. All too often caregivers are dealing with issues not yet fully or satisfactorily researched and understood scientifically. Doctors, nurses, and dentists must be able to walk the fine line between telling it like it is to the patient and doing what they know to be of some assistance in reducing the pattern of self-destructive behavior. In my own experience, I have failed to appreciate the possibility of serious alcohol or other drug addiction at times when I could have made a difference to those afflicted.

I have also learned to try to approach every patient, and in the end, everyone, in a nonjudgmental manner. In this way I seek to realize Leston Havens's vision, discussed earlier, of occupying the same space with that other person, without feeling the need either to invade or be invaded by the other. I think it helps in dealing with patients or those who are suffering.

Mass Media and Desensitization

Television, movies, electronic games, novels, comic books, and even the evening news are so full of violence and death that it is rare to go through a day without viewing or hearing about some horribly violent or disturbing event. Explicit movies illustrate how to kill, injure, or mutilate others or oneself, and the media makes major figures of many of the sorriest examples of human degradation. Modern-day casualness toward killing and death makes it easier and easier to minimize respect for life and harder and harder to empathize with others who are suffering in some significant way. Almost as much as they feature violence, mass media tend to focus on the mundane, the material, the quick fix, the one time around, leaving unaddressed the real suffering lurking in the background.

Another way in which the media can affect our relationship to suffering is through their love affair with wealth, fame, youth, beauty, perfection, and celebrity. Suffering, pain, and adjustment to adversity can seem to be foreign substances in the mainstream recipe for the good life. Moreover, when suffering is portrayed in popular entertainment, it is usually short-lived and often resolved in a fortunate turn of events. This is not to say there are not many psychologically constructive and socially useful depictions through the arts of the true nature of suffering. Aristotle believed that tragedy served an important therapeutic function because of the emotional catharsis it engendered in the audience. There are many modern examples of what Aristotle meant. And of course we cannot simply blame the media for presenting what we either want or are willing to buy. But in terms of the issue at hand, we need only look at the media to see the good, bad, and neutral in our cultural perceptions of suffering.

Desensitization to suffering can also occur within the health care setting. Overloaded urban emergency rooms provide an example of a situation in which suffering becomes so commonplace that caregivers' emotional responses can easily begin to shut down. Health care providers in general, regardless of their particular work setting, run the risk of becoming desensitized to suffering. These circumstances illustrate a tension inherent in the provision of health care between the importance of being efficient, objective, analytical, and to a certain degree dispassionate and the importance of recognizing suffering, feeling compassion, and expressing empathy to those who suffer.

Reductionist View of Medicine

The Newtonian, reductionist, biomolecular orientation of modern physicianhood emphasizes scientific intervention through its focus on disease's molecular causes and therapies. Consequently, it has little to do with such things as the healing relationship. Some decades ago, Donald Seldin, a wonderfully gifted physician-scientist, opined that the needs and opportunities for molecular medicine were so great that the leaders of scientific medicine should focus their energies on the pursuit of diseases in terms of their molecular causes and therapies, leaving the psyches and personalities, wants and needs, hopes and fears, social problems and familial relationships of patients in the domain of nurses and social workers.[13]

Arthur Kleinman perceives this orientation to be somewhat built into our society's view of illness. He writes:

> Social reality is so organized that we do not routinely inquire into the meanings of illness any more than we regularly analyze the structure of our social world. Indeed, the everyday priority structure of medical training and of health care delivery, with its radically materialistic pursuit of the biological mechanism of disease, precludes such inquiry. It turns the gaze of the clinician, along with the attention of patients and families, away from decoding the salient meanings of illness for them, which interferes with recognition of disturbing but potentially treatable problems in their life world. The biomedical system replaces this allegedly "soft," therefore devalued, psychosocial concern with meanings, with

the scientifically "hard," therefore overvalued, technical quest for the control of symptoms. This pernicious value transformation is a serious failing of modern medicine: it disables the healer and dis-empowers the chronically ill."[14]

I have for many years focused critically upon Donald Seldin's opinion on this matter, in part because I was oriented to contesting his view in the minds of physicians seeking to grow in their professional lives. With specialization's increasing expansion of the health care team, perhaps we should accept Seldin's view as expressing an aspect of reality. We can make use of it as appropriate in asserting that the health care team must provide the necessary human support for patient and family, as well as the appropriate biomedical intervention. I think all doctors must become aware of these matters. If they are too busy to tend to these matters, they should care enough to see to it that, if at all possible, their patients have the necessary support systems in place.

Perhaps the most provocative and compelling of all the truly exceptional books on human suffering is *The Patient's Ordeal* by William May. The first striking thing about this book is Professor May's approach to the subject. He devotes his first eight chapters respectively to "the burned . . . the retarded . . . the retarded institutionalized . . . the gestated and sold . . . the battered . . . the molested . . . the aged, their virtues and vices . . . [and] afflicting the afflicted—total institutions."[15] His last two chapters describe how the afflicted assist the afflicted; for example, in Alcoholics Anonymous and through organ donations for transplants.

I have read this book several times since it was published in 1991, because it provides important and sometimes arresting insights into the extreme and particular sufferings of various groups of people. Even for those of us who have experienced life-threatening illnesses, it is important to remember, and to remind others, about the nature and extraordinary degree of largely unnoticed emotional and physical suffering that often accompanies serious illness. Professor May's approach motivates the reader to want to work on reducing the isolation and desolation of such people.

Likewise, Kleinman illuminates the important distinction between a disease, which may well be diagnosed and treated at a molecular level, and the associated illness, which affects the whole of the patient's life and requires a broader perspective for therapeutic support. If suffering is in fact a sense of impending personal disintegration, then clearly the reductionist physician Seldin describes is not of a mind to participate in relieving emotional suffering or likely to be concerned with understanding or even recognizing it. Kleinman's view of the "technical quest for control of symptoms" points to a similar circumstance. The bottom-line message to patients and to society is one of exclusion from the purview of modern medicine and its high priests, those we have cloaked with the vestments associated with marrying advanced technology to humanity. Suffering—social and psychological pain—is simply not part of the equation.

What Can We Do?

One thing that we can do was called to my attention by Dr. Lawrence Tancredi, a psychiatrist colleague who reviewed an early draft of this chapter and counseled me on the subject. When I joined the Institute of Medicine as the second employee and deputy to the president, one of my tasks was to develop a plan for the senior staff member we needed to acquire in the first year or two. As it became clear that we wanted someone with credentials and experience in the ethical and human values dimensions of health and health care, we found and recruited Larry Tancredi, then a young psychiatrist-lawyer. Later, when I became president of the University of Texas

Health Science Center at Houston, he was one of four individuals my colleagues and I recruited to the campus to serve as university professors and teach in all six of our health professional schools. I learned to seek his opinion on many issues and have come to trust his insights.

Regarding this chapter, Dr. Tancredi encouraged me to include a section on the benefits that may be associated with suffering. Upon reflection, I can come up with four possible benefits from my own experience, some of which other patients might wish to consider. First is the anxiety reduction that comes from having "been there, done that," from having suffered and survived the experience without being broken by it. Second was the somewhat unexpected sense of community with others who have traveled and may still be traveling a similar path. I have always felt that suffering is connected to one's natural fear of dying. As with dying, unavoidable suffering is for each individual a significant life challenge that both tests and rewards our human capacity to adapt and endure.

The third and fourth positives are creativity and spiritual growth. I am far from alone among patients with chronic diseases who have found great satisfaction in drawing and painting. Although I may be repeating myself here, the very fact of having had a close encounter with the end of life has been a stimulus for me to further try to penetrate the spiritual dimension of my life. It is partly why I have returned to reading some of Thomas Merton's writings. It is also related to, but more than, Samuel Johnson's famous saying, "[W]hen a man knows he is to be hanged in a fortnight, it concentrates his mind wonderfully."

Dr. Tancredi wrote to me about this as follows:

One thought that hit me was the interesting literature on suffering and creativity, a literature that includes the role of manic depression, and depression (plus suicide) and the creative process, but also an underlying notion that in suffering there is a nearly dispassionate separation of things sensual, body from mind and emotions, thereby freeing one up so to speak for a creative effort. This is seen most explicitly in Mann's *The Magic Mountain*, where consumption of the body seems related to enhancement of the soul and mind. Also one is impressed by the number of great writers who not only suffered from psychological illnesses but physical ones as well . . . I recognize that you are focusing on one view of suffering, but the enhancing aspects (the belief that suffering is purification and not just punishment, and is essential for personal elevation) have been basic to the monastic tradition and continue in the tradition of many literary works as well.

There is more that one could say and others who can shed light in this area, but the essential point is that, when suffering finds us, potentially positive dimensions may come with the experience.

If one asks the question, Is society insensitive to suffering? the immediate answers are unsatisfying. So far in this discussion, we have been emphasizing the various ways in which society denies, misinterprets, and even promotes suffering. On the other hand, ours is a society that spends more money than any other on the care of the sick. We have done as much or more than other nations to include the disabled in our public and private systems; the Americans for Disabilities Act of 1990 signified our nation's commitment to fully integrating those with disabilities into American life. We have also brought about some of the world's most sweeping changes in disease prevention through smoking bans, lower, safer speed limits, and environmental regulation. Critics could properly comment that each of these positive initiatives is flawed in terms of incorporating suffering creatively into our national life. Nevertheless, we are doing some things well.

Thus society, although not completely insensitive to suffering, could definitely enhance our personal and institutional sensibilities concerning suffering. Mindful of how difficult and complicated it will be for society to achieve this, I nonetheless offer some suggestions.

First, we need more discussion about suffering and its meaning in our individual lives and in our culture (as Gilpin Faust has reminded us in her history of suffering and death in the American Civil War). As a nation of optimists, expansionists, and youth and beauty idolaters, we shrink from thinking of life as a dance with illness and death. Talking and thinking about suffering are important steps in removing the taboos surrounding it and recognizing that it is part of the human condition and the community. The myth that suffering is avoidable needs to be reshaped to include it in the inescapable stuff of life. Suffering is something we can work to minimize and seek to prevent wherever possible, but we cannot completely eliminate it from our lives. Suffering, which is shared by all of us, could be an uniting force among us rather than something divisive and alienating. Each of us needs to be seeking out friends who are suffering, rather than subconsciously ignoring them or their suffering. Acknowledging suffering does not make it go away, but it lessens the painful isolation that it so often imposes on those it afflicts.

Second, our society needs to integrate its traditional values in a less superficial understanding of individuality and hope for a long, pain-free, blemish-free existence, unencumbered by the responsibilities of social ties. It is true and good that our progress in the treatment of pain has led to the subsequent reduction of some incapacities associated with chronic disease. But we have overemphasized self-sufficiency. We cannot continue to neglect our own and others' need for community, especially in dealing with illness and suffering.

Health care providers, by virtue of their closeness to suffering, are in a position to apply the above approaches where they are most likely to have significant impact. Moreover, the nature of the responsibility to treat illness implies attention to suffering, which some refer to "as the hidden dimension of illness."[16] The social, psychological, and even religious spheres from which some suffering emanates do as much to define what it means to be ill as genetic aberrations and physiological malfunctions. Just as health care providers endeavor, in the interest of healing, to uncover the physical origins of disease, they should try for the same reason to discover and address the fuller panoply of concerns associated with illness.

For health care providers, the first step in addressing suffering may be to expand their usual focus to incorporate the emotional, aesthetic, and human dimensions of personality. The "Seldin solution" referred to earlier should be replaced with a broader view of science and healing and of the border between the science and art of medicine. Science does seem to be moving in this direction. More and more biomedical scientists are beginning to agree that expanding the paradigm beyond Newtonian concepts should not compromise their ability to mine reductionist theory for as yet undiscovered treasure.[17] This movement in biomedicine—partly because of its insistence that the scientist-observer cannot be considered an external observer, but is part of the experiment or experience—may help to restore behavioral science to full intellectual partnership in the academic health science community. Movement in this direction will also serve to expand awareness of the importance of dealing constructively and openly with suffering within the scientific enterprise.

Clinicians and patients alike would do well to educate themselves about suffering. The volume of literature in this area is small but growing, as the impact of the social context of illness becomes better appreciated. AIDS has opened up national and international discussion of suffering, which has helped demystify the subject. In particular, the AIDS literature written by patients themselves has much to teach about suffering. Those who have studied suffering have observed common phenomena of which every clinician should be aware. One of the lessons here is that the degree of suffering one experiences has little to do with the intensity of physical pain. Equally valuable is the observation that suffering is often masked by apathy; and that apathy often reflects hopelessness and not, for example, a lack of motivation to get better. On the other hand, it is well to remember that our technical advances in controlling and preventing pain do serve to reduce suffering and often make possible therapeutic and diagnostic interventions otherwise not approachable.

As much as health care workers should be aware of what is known about suffering, they should take stock of their own biases and consider how these may color their perceptions of patients and their suffering. One might question one's underlying beliefs about suffering. Is it divine punishment for transgressions? Does it signify personal weakness? For example, perhaps negative childhood experiences with an alcoholic parent have made one unsympathetic to the suffering of the addicted. Or perhaps one's upbringing has produced a simplistic view of the suffering of other ethnic or racial groups. Some may have a high tolerance for pain or for solitude, and may therefore be at risk of discounting the potential of such stimuli to elicit suffering in others. Understanding the lenses through which we view the world can help us more clearly discern the nature of the images we see through those lenses. Needless to say, the more we as caregivers learn about these things, the better equipped we will be to assist our patients in their difficult times. Likewise, the more we know about these matters as patients, the better we will function as board chairs of our health care teams and rally our capacity for self-healing.

In a similar vein, caregivers must also monitor how their physical and emotional energy levels affect their interactions with patients and their capacity to recognize and respond compassionately to suffering and illness. The overcrowded and chaotic urban emergency room is a salient example of a setting where desensitization and "burn-out" may prevent clinicians from recognizing suffering in others. The importance of taking time for self-renewal cannot be overemphasized; frustration and exhaustion can easily overwhelm compassion.

Institutional environments may also complicate the recognition and management of suffering. The machines of medicine whirring and beeping not only focus medical staff's attention on the physiologic processes of disease—respiration, heartbeat, blood pressure, and the like—but also may intimidate patients and their families as they try to contemplate illness, loss, and perhaps even death. Providers should seek to minimize the negative impacts of such environmental factors, to make time and space for the low-tech, less tangible aspects of care to occur.

Where for whatever reason practitioners find it difficult or impossible to ameliorate a patient's emotional suffering, they should be aware of other resources—counselors, clergy, support groups, community activities—with which the patient can be connected. As clinicians keep up on biomedical advances, they should also remember these sorts of interventions.

In the effort to energize an effective change in group or organizational behavior, it is often valuable to have the backing of interested, but uninvolved, outside groups, foundations, or commissions. One of the most important foundation-supported efforts to humanize modern patient care has been the Picker-Commonwealth Program, begun in 1987, to identify the elements and promote the development of patient-centered care. This program approaches health care from the perspective of the patient rather than the convenience or interests of health care providers. A comprehensive review of what the program uncovered and learned is contained in a volume published in 1993, authored by the researchers and physicians who led much of that effort. Entitled *Through the Patient's Eyes: Understanding and Promoting*

Patient-Centered Care, it lays out a comprehensive blueprint for a more humane health care approach, including provision of curing, caring and preventive services.[18]

Probably the most overlooked powerful tool for handling suffering is communication. It sounds so simple: ask patients if they are suffering. But many clinicians don't do it. Or perhaps they don't engage in the conversation in the most effective way. Often the understanding and alleviation of suffering require communication at a different level—communication about the significance of an illness in an individual's life. Is the patient who has had hip replacement surgery an active person who gets great pleasure from physical activity and independence? Could weeks of inactivity and dependence upon caregivers precipitate a depression? Perhaps hip replacement surgery preceded the rapid decline of a parent's health or a friend's participation in shared activities. The bottom line is that an inquiry into the current suffering, if any, on the part of the patient should be at the top of any caregiver's to-do list.

Often a patient's suffering and other health issues do not have a cut-and-dried solution, but can be treated in various ways, each with its pluses and minuses. Internist John Santo has recently offered an admirable model of how to present such options to patients and empower them to decide how to proceed. Dr. Santo gives examples from his own practice, in which he impartially presented patients and their families with acceptable and reasonable options for care, including each option's risks and benefits. The patients and their families often chose differently from what he expected, based on his prior knowledge of them. But what surprised him even more was that even when a treatment option did not turn out well, he was not blamed. Instead, the patient and family appreciated their decision-making role. According to Dr. Santo, "Our relationship remained strong until [the patient's] death, largely because she, not someone else, remained in control of her treatment."[19] Focusing on respecting patients' need to keep in control of their lives seems to me a constructive way to help them manage their suffering.

Likewise, Howard Brody has pointed out that suffering increases when patients feel they are not respected by caregivers and others around them.[20] Physicians and other caregivers must at the very least show their patients that they value and respect them as members of the community. Such efforts obviously become more difficult when health care teams do not reflect the racial and ethnic diversity of the patient communities they serve. This is one of the most important reasons why the ranks of physicians and other caregivers should continue to become less homogenous than they have traditionally been. By discussing and considering these issues—even if we don't collectively reach the same conclusions—we can contribute to America's emotional, intellectual, and spiritual growth as we address suffering as well as joy, illness as well as health, and death as well as life. Future healers may find that these issues are absolutely crucial to their development, and possibly to their patients' health as well.

Chapter 5

Where Life and Death Meet

In 1960, nearing the end of medical school, I wrote in the *Harvard Medical Bulletin*:

There was a soft gurgle followed by a gush of clear fluid that poured out of her mouth and onto her chest.

She's dead, I thought. My first death.

The intern, in his second week at the Boston City Hospital, rushed off confusedly to try to do something about it. She was his patient. She was dead. I was a fourth year medical student and had no ultimate responsibility, and actually accepted the fact of her death minutes before he did. It was an awesome experience—I had finally witnessed that against which all medicine is aimed. Like most of us, I wanted never to lose my respect and sense of awe for death. I vowed that at each subsequent deathbed I would recall, or try to recall, some of the feelings that moved me this first time.

One week later, we rushed down the ward to the bedside of an apneic, cyanotic, cardiac patient, aged 65. An intern was thumping the patient's chest. I tried to figure out what I would do next were I the intern. The epinephrine was injected into the patient's heart. I was waiting and hoping for my first open thoracotomy at this, my third deathbed. But the intern decided against it. I was disappointed. The patient's heart had stopped. If he had held out a few minutes longer, there might have been a thoracotomy. Another student ran out to get an ophthalmoscope in order to try and see what was happening in the fundi at the hour of death. My interest picked up again. He returned and looked in. Zealously, in my turn, I pulled back the dead lid, satisfied in my pursuit of knowledge, happy with my intellectual curiosity, focused the ophthalmoscope and saw, realized, remembered what I was doing.

The awareness at this time of the obvious defect in my attitude and my perplexity over how to repair it brought to mind the somewhat curious statement made to me five years before by a practicing internist who said that one of the most startling, humbling, yet exciting aspects of the practice of medicine for him was to be with, and to somehow try to help, patients who, with their backs against the wall, finally turned around to confront death.

It is a curious fact that we as future physicians spend countless hours learning about life, how to preserve it, and learning about diseases, how they can kill; and yet, we avoid thinking about death as well as the next person. Surely, we are young, we have not really entertained the thought of not being. Nevertheless, it seems appropriate that we, in some senses, should be the experts about death, and that we not misinterpret that 11th medical commandment, which says, "Thou shalt not get emotionally involved with your patients."

Our society, rightly or wrongly, for better or for worse,

predisposes us to the position that death is the ultimate evil—
the thing to be avoided at all costs.[1]

Witnessing death for the first time creates vivid images, and my
recollection of that event remains with me to this day. No doubt it is
much the same with any medical student's—indeed, any person's—
first experience with death.

The tenet that doctors not get emotionally involved with their
patients is also still with us, as is the belief that the point of medicine
is to delay if not defeat death. But the winds of change, or at least
gusts here and there, have appeared. In the past two decades much
progress has been made in the care of the terminally ill. But some issues remain for both patients and clinicians.

Let's continue with my words of 1960 and see if they still reflect
aspects of medicine today.

It is obviously crucial to teach medical students the intrica-
cies of every method or technique that might possibly bring
someone back from extremis. It is vital that no potential life-
saving step be overlooked, but it does seem somewhat symptomatic that few words, if any, have ever been spoken to us
about how to help persons die. It is our duty to see that they
die "in balance" [that is, without unbalanced blood
chemistries indicating a correctable problem] but no one has
ever suggested that we ought to make an attempt to care for
their psyches during their last hours. We all believe that it is
poor medicine not to "treat the whole patient" and furthermore we will expend a great deal of energy in enhancing their
physical comfort in small ways, which may have no influence
on the final outcome of their sickness—and yet it is not
always noticed that dying patients very often seem to
have less attention paid to them than to the patency of the

multiplicity of tubes that are entering them from every direction, and which will enable us to study posthumously the last, hopefully balanced, chemistries. It is not always noticed that more real effort is expended to get autopsy permission than to see to it that the patient does not die alone. It is almost as though, as doctors, we express our denial of death by focusing our attention upon the tubes, the chemistries, and the autopsy.

We tend to regard our treatment as having failed if the patient dies. "Successful treatment" is a term too often reserved only for those who live. One could submit another category, that of the successfully treated terminal event. One could suggest that the physicians throw off their scientific mantle when at the deathbed, and become something else— and that something ought to be whatever the patient requires. It is apparent that, for physicians in modern America to do this, they must be capable of dealing sympathetically with agnostic, atheist, Protestant, Jew, Moslem, or Catholic, with what they may consider personally to be unreasonable, superstition, or sheer lunacy. It is hard for a student to talk about this ability in a physician because it seems that experience, both external and internal as well as sincere effort are needed before one can succeed in becoming expert (if indeed one ever can) at helping the dying person through death. Here, if anywhere, is the greatest stronghold of the practice of the art of medicine; here, as in every other area of medicine, is what one accomplishes proportional to what one offers; here, too, is what one offers proportional to what one knows.

Now, let's fast-forward fifty years to one of the most compelling explications of the "American way of death" and its potential for inflicting a drawn-out dying time with unnecessary indignities, suffering, and loss of independence for the patient. Describing his practice as an internist in a large hospital, Dr. Craig Bowron says:

> I see adult patients of all ages and complexities, most of whom make good recoveries and return to life as they knew it. But taking care of the threadbare elderly, those facing an eternal winter with no green in sight, is definitely the most difficult thing I do. That's because never before in history has it been so hard to fulfill our final earthly task: Dying. It used to be that people were visited by death. With nothing to fight it, we simply accepted it and grieved. Today, thanks to myriad medications and interventions that have been created to improve our health and prolong our lives, dying has become a difficult and often excruciatingly slow process."[2]

Dr. Bowron then presents three case examples of the problems faced today by aged patients, their families, and their caregivers. One patient is an eighty-five-year-old woman with complex chronic diseases, who for six months has been on dialysis and is largely demented. She spends three days of every week hooked up to a dialysis machine and the other four days recovering from the dialysis. Her family has kept her on "full code," meaning do everything possible to resuscitate her if she suddenly stops breathing or goes into shock.

The second story is of a ninety-one-year-old man with problems of daily nursing care of a greater magnitude than any Dr. Bowron had seen before. The doctor was stunned to find out that this man was being taken care of at his home, by his son—alone. The son, a Vietnam veteran, devoted his entire life to his father's care.

The third patient was eighty-six years old and came to the hospital from a nursing home with her diabetes out of control. She had serious dementia, a broken hip, pneumonia, and other complications.

When the doctor spoke with the patient's son about setting a code status of "do not resuscitate" (DNR), the son said she should never have been brought to the hospital in the first place because, at his mother's explicit request, he and his siblings had several years ago agreed to DNR status. Once again, they chose the DNR order for their mother.

Dr. Bowron follows these three case presentations with important observations about the caregivers of such threadbare elderly and dying patients:

> To be clear: Everyone dies. There are no life-saving medications, only life-prolonging ones. To say that anyone chooses to die is, in most situations, a misstatement of the facts. But medical advances have created at least the façade of choice. It appears as if death has made a counter-offer and that the responsibility is now ours.
>
> In today's world, an elderly person or their family must "choose," for example, between dialysis and death, or a feeding tube and death. Those can be very simple choices when you're 40 and critically ill; they can be agonizing when you're 80 and the bad days outnumber the good days two to one.
>
> It's not hard to identify one of these difficult cases in the hospital. Among the patient-care team—nurses, physicians, nursing assistants, physical and occupational therapists, etc.— there is often a palpable sense of "What in the world are we doing to this patient?" That's "to" and not "for." We all stagger under the weight of feeling complicit in a patient's torture, but often it's the nurses who bear most of the burden, physically and emotionally. As a nurse on a dialysis floor told me, "They'll tell us things that they won't tell the family or their physician. They'll say, 'I don't want to have any more dialysis. I'm tired of it,' but they won't admit that to anyone else."

This sense of complicity is what makes taking care of these kinds of patients the toughest thing I do. A fellow physician told me, "I feel like I am participating in something immoral." Another asked, "Whatever happened to that 'do no harm' business?"[3]

Dr. Bowron's examples of what we may call "overtreatment" illustrate the extraordinary suffering it can inflict on patients, their families, and even their caregivers. They also show how the cause of overtreatment may be the family's desire not to let go or glitches in the system, such as nursing home personnel's failure to recognize the DNR code on a patient's records. Sadly, there is also often an equally understandable but less excusable factor: money.

A physician friend, now in a nephrology private practice, took his kidney specialty training in a major medical center that exposed him for considerable periods of time to patients in three hospital settings: a large, public, mostly Medicaid/Medicare–funded hospital; a Veterans Hospital; and a large hospital catering to private paying clientele, almost all of whom had excellent insurance coverage, including Medicare. During a two-year experience in the 1990s, he noted that when it came to the patients at the end of their long lives, there was a clear difference between the patterns of care in the two public hospitals and in the private hospital. His observation was a rather astounding paradox: there was a better capacity in the public hospitals to let the terminal patients pass away without dramatic interventions, such as dialysis, than in the private hospital. In the latter circumstances, he personally felt, as did some nursing staff, a diminution of morale over continuing these apparently hopeless patients on dialysis for an unnecessarily extended hospital stay until death supervened. As a trainee, he saw this behavior as the attending physicians' responses to the financial incentives to provide more care.

It could also be true that patients' families might have been playing a role, at least some of the time, in not stopping care that had become futile. But I thought of my friend's experiences in that particular hospital when a prominent lawyer—a former board member at that hospital and leading opinion maker in the city—more or less accosted me after a public evening talk I had given on the subject of death and dying. On his way out, he shook my hand with his right hand while grabbing my tie at the collar with his left hand and said, "It is your moral obligation to teach doctors to let old people die in peace."

For decades the Dartmouth Atlas of Health Care has been mapping health care practice variations and associated cost and quality measures, under the direction of John Wennberg and Eliot Fisher. Its findings have consistently shown a two- to threefold variation in the cost of care for the elderly; for example, between Minneapolis and Miami. Along with much other evidence, the Dartmouth Atlas indicates that physician practice habits are conditioned by the paradoxical financial incentives encouraging more high-tech treatment. This situation is especially problematic for the frail elderly and their families, if their general aim is usually to live and to die as comfortably as possible.

There is no perfect answer to every such case. However, there is little question that patient choices regarding major therapeutic interventions are very often more conservative than the possibilities offered by caregivers. We know this to be true for such things as breast surgery, treatment for benign prostatic hypertrophy, and an increasing list of interventions. By "conservative" I mean times when the patient has two choices for dealing with a particular problem: typically surgical intervention, or a medical or pharmaceutical treatment combined with watchful waiting. For example, in the case of many patients with significant and symptomatic benign prostatic enlargement, the most conservative choice would be watchful waiting and the most interventionist would be surgery.

We also know from the Dartmouth group that when academic physicians were faced with similar symptoms and were equally informed by the same specialist physicians of their options, some chose surgery and some chose the conservative approach. The outcomes were equally satisfactory from the patients' points of view. In these areas where choice is required, cost and the inconvenience and suffering of a treatment must be considered. Inevitably, doctors' incentives enter into the calculus. It is important to remember that, at least until the current housing credit crisis and recession occurred, health care debt caused more than 60 percent of personal bankruptcy cases in the United States!

The same reasoning may also apply for what is reasonable treatment for the frail elderly clearly facing death in the near term. In June 1960 I entered my internship and residency in internal medicine at the University of Washington. There Dr. Belding Scribner was implementing the first chronic hemodialysis program in the world, for patients who would otherwise die in renal failure. Which patients should get this scarce resource? The original few patients were the path breakers. Once their survival was documented, Dr. Scribner concluded that he shouldn't be the gatekeeper for these limited resources. Thus, an autonomous committee of citizens (*Time* magazine labeled this "the God Committee") was set up to choose who would be accepted into the program. Over the next few years, doctors could refer people from King County, Washington, for consideration for what was then a hospital-based hemodialysis program. Since there were only a few dialysis machines, there were very few available openings for new patients.

Although this approach received various criticisms at the time from ethicists, critics, and commentators around the country, many of us working in that exciting but challenging environment accepted that we as physicians could only build our best medical case for our patients. An independent and anonymous group made the decisions as to acceptance into the program when an opening developed. Over the next decade, we all saw several lives saved by this scarce resource, but we also saw how many others might have been saved. As time went on, more patients were successfully treated with a slowly growing number of dialysis machines. By 1972, social and political pressure built to the point that the Seattle-based nephrologists dialyzed one of their original patients, then ten years after his original dialysis, in front of Chairman Wilbur Mills and the Congressional Budget Committee. Within days, Mills's committee approved legislation adding Medicare coverage for treatment for patients with renal failure at any age.

Early in the 1960s, I was one of the medical team caring for the middle-aged wife of a physician from Spokane, Washington. She had acute renal failure and had dialysis long enough to show that her kidneys would never recover. By that time arrangements had been made to admit patients to the program from parts of Washington outside King County. As her medical evaluation wore on, we hoped she would be chosen for the chronic dialysis program. When she was, we were all elated. But to our astonishment, after a couple of days of consultation with her husband and children, she decided she didn't want to live so much of her life tied to such a cumbersome machine.

At that time dialysis was in its infancy. Using the process as a permanent treatment was a forbidding prospect, but I don't believe anyone had previously rejected the possibility. After the woman was dialyzed for the last time, she left for Spokane looking quite fit—to face certain death within a few weeks. She impressed me as one of the most mature people I had ever met, and the provocative implications of her decision a half century ago are still with me. Although kidney transplantation might have been on the horizon, I have no doubt that her decision was the correct one for her, even though none of us caregivers believed she would pass up what we saw as breakthrough treatment. The caregiver's role is to correctly present the viable options to the patient, who in this case acted decisively and effectively as the de facto chair of her own medical and health board.

During this period, just as the age of hypertechnology in medicine was gaining momentum, Pope Pius XII declared that there was no moral imperative to use artificial means of any sort to treat the otherwise dying patient, other than what we now refer to as "comfort care." I remember the impact and influence this statement had on doctors and nurses of all faiths, and no faith. It meant that external respirators, renal dialysis, cardiopulmonary respiratory techniques, and other exciting new advances were not required to be used in hopeless situations. Nevertheless, whenever such a situation occurred and led to a decision not to go further with extraordinary treatments, it was hard on everyone involved.

At the time, the decision to end treatment was a medical one. Then it became a bureaucratic one. Today, perhaps appropriately in our litigious culture, such decisions are wrapped in legal trappings, with the fear of lawsuits and accusations of malpractice always present. However, I believe there is a common sense, universal wisdom in Pope Pius XII's appeal that can still form the basis of a mature cultural outlook on the terminally ill in this county. This view respects a patient's decision not to get chronic dialysis or a heart transplant to survive. Right now, society can insist that a life-saving treatment be given to a child in a family whose religious beliefs forbid such interventions, but we do not impose life-saving treatments on independent adults against their will. This is as it should be.

It is useful and good for patients to know that only fifty years ago, American culture was not known for incorporating death into life. More often it was denied or treated as a tragedy. Medical students of the midtwentieth century were foremost among the "death-denying personalities," seemingly preselected by their ambition to defeat death. Dr. Elizabeth Kübler-Ross and Dame Cicely Saunders, who founded the hospice movement, did much over the past four decades to create a healthier environment for patients, families, and caregivers alike.

Solving the Riddle

The twenty-first century has produced such amazing technical advances that we seem to be able to follow the patient's molecular status virtually by the minute. Consequently, the need to do an autopsy on every patient has been significantly reduced. Although there are good reasons (cost benefit among them) for this fairly major reduction in the rate of autopsies, studies show that more often than one would like, autopsies reveal mistaken diagnoses and treatments. The routinely held, old-fashioned death conferences to review every death in the hospital with the clinical story to be told, punctuated by the postmortem findings of the examining pathologist, were the ultimate quality of care assessment tool.

In some senses, the death of a patient is viewed as an insult or setback to us as physicians; it means we may have failed in our duty. A successfully treated patient is a healthy patient. The most extreme example of an unsuccessfully treated patient is a patient no longer alive. In his book *How We Die*, Sherwin Nuland considers what may underlie this perception. He writes:

> Doctors are people who succeed—that is how they survived the fierce competition to achieve their medical degree, their training, and their position. Like other talented people, they require constant reassurance of their abilities.[4]

Feelings of failure when a dying patient cannot be saved may be responsible for the "wounded healer" syndrome. Doctors as a group suffer from stress far more than most other members of society and are more likely to have problems with chemical dependencies. Surgeon Bernie Siegel writes in his bestselling book *Love, Medicine, and Miracles*:

> Throughout our training we learn *not* to empathize with the sick, supposedly to save us psychic strain … The emotional distance hurts both parties, however. We withdraw just when patients need us most. Nurses know how hard it is to find a doctor when a patient is dying. All our education encourages us to think of ourselves as gods of repair, miracle workers. When we can't fix what's broken, we crawl off to lick our wounds, feeling like failures. The distance also encourages doctors to feel invulnerable: "It's always other people who are sick, not me." When I tell a roomful of medical students, "Almost everybody dies," they all laugh; but when I say the same line to a roomful of doctors, there's dead silence. We become the best deniers of all.[5]

In the past three decades, medical science has come up with more advanced ways to keep alive many people on the brink of death. The idea that doctors should try everything to keep the patient alive is pervasive, even if being alive entails further agony as inevitable death is prolonged. Our increasing control over the timing or occurrence of death obviously has positive implications for patients who are able to return to lives of quality, but it can also bring about frightening, painful, and prolonged deaths. Our technology has in many cases outpaced our spiritual understanding of death as well as our compassion for dying patients. In addition, the environment for malpractice in our litigious society may motivate doctors to pursue every method of sustaining life in these impossible situations, even when that course of action may be harmful to themselves and patients alike. On the other hand, it is sometimes impossible to know what the odds of an unusual recovery are in any particular situation. Nuland describes the dilemma posed by the almost endless array of technological treatment options:

> Pursuing treatment against great odds may seem like a heroic act to some, but too commonly it is a form of unwilling disservice to patients; it blurs the borders of candor and reveals a fundamental schism between the best interests of patients and their families on the one hand and of physicians on the other.[6]

Timothy Quill, in *Death and Dignity: Making Choices and Taking Charge,* writes of this dilemma:

> When the possibility for meaningful recovery becomes remote, then burdensome treatment begins to feel more like torture than a difficult means to a higher purpose. If the decision makers successfully shield themselves from the true burdens of treatment or from the reality that a patient is dying, then medical treatment can unintentionally prolong and dehumanize the dying process.[7]

It is not always clear when imminent death is inevitable. But just as Edmund Pellegrino, the distinguished physician-philosopher, has long advocated that the physician should never become the purposeful agent of death, he also strongly emphasizes the role of the physician in reducing pain and suffering. Aggressive treatment in the face of inevitable death may wrongly give patients and their families false hopes, or "cheat" them out of a more peaceful parting. In addition, as Craig Bowron and others have testified, it can also be demoralizing to physicians and other health care providers.

Nuland defines the drive that many physicians experience to

understand the precise details of a patient's pathophysiology, to make a diagnosis, and to design and carry out a specific cure—sometimes without regard to the well-being of the patient—as "solving The Riddle." He writes:

> The satisfaction of solving The Riddle is its own reward, and the fuel that drives the clinical engines of medicine's most highly trained specialists. It is every doctor's measure of his own abilities; it is the most important ingredient in his professional self image . . . A physician's driving quest to solve The Riddle will sometimes be at odds with our best interests at the end of life.[8]

Societal and patient perceptions of doctors can also energize the quest to solve "The Riddle." People tend to believe that doctors' reasons for recommending certain courses of action are wholly scientific. It is easy to overlook other motivational factors that may be at play in doctors' medical decision making, such as the need to preserve their own image as conquerors of disease and the perverse financial incentives in our fragmented health care scene. All is not lost, however, even if we can't find the energy to fix our system. Many health professionals march to different drummers than financial ones. As Dr. Harvey Minchew points out in his introduction to this book, the best physicians are driven not so much to solve The Riddle as to solve the patients' problems. In fact, in working with him closely and following how he handled patients I referred to him, I can attest that his intellect was not focused on any interesting riddle but was driven specifically toward puzzles central to his patients' problems, distress, and health status.

Let's continue with my words from 1960:

It is clear that we ought to be familiar with the concept that death is a cruel and utter end to some people, while only a transition to something better or worse to others, and that we ought to be willing to act accordingly in our relationships with our patients. It is also obvious that any consideration of death does become philosophical and theological, and is therefore rather subjective. But there must be something more we can know, objectively, collectively, to sharpen our sensibilities, deepen our insight, broaden our background, and thus enhance our understanding of any given patient in his last hours.

Operating on this premise, I thumbed through the Widener Library card catalogue labeled "Death," and found that death has meant different things to different people and to different cultures, that rites and rituals, myths and symbols have grown up around the terminal event and that an understanding of these varying attitudes is both interesting and revealing.[9]

Evolving Perceptions of Death

In 1960 the card catalogue of Harvard University's Widener Library yielded almost solely literary, artistic, and anthropologic treatments of the subject of death. Over the past few decades, however, many medical and sociological researchers have turned their attention to it. For example, Daniel Callahan's *The Troubled Dream of Life* provides an interesting historical account of evolving perceptions of death. Callahan's book relates how death used to be more familiar, a steady and routine part of daily life. Death frequently took place in the home, amid family and friends who gathered to give meaning to the dying person's final moments and show communal solidarity in the face of death. Prior to the rise of scientific medicine in the eighteenth century, medicine could do little to alter the course of critical illness, and death from illness was an openly accepted part of life.[10]

With scientific medicine came new drugs, new tools, new treatments, and increased life expectancy. New beliefs about death also began to take shape. People no longer saw death as a fixed, collective destiny but as a personal tragedy to be prevented, or at least delayed. Where death was once a "public" event, it now became private and somehow negative or even shameful. People felt the need to sanitize the experience of death. Families began to take their dying relatives to hospitals and nursing homes to die. Presuming that ignorance was bliss, doctors often lied to dying patients to spare them an agonizing anticipation of death. And in society, death became a topic that was simply not discussed.

Although we have begun to explore the meaning of death in our modern society, and to wonder whether we have perhaps made coping with it more difficult by shrouding it in secrecy, we have yet to fully integrate death into our collective psyche, despite its inevitability. Callahan writes:

> Death has not come out of the closet, only its foot is showing ... For all of its great triumphs, contemporary medicine does not know what to make of death. The end of life represents a troubling, and particularly recent, vacuum in its thinking. Death has no well-understood place in medical theory, even if it remains omnipresent in practice. There is a "presumption to treat" in medical care that protects physicians if they initiate emergency, potentially life-saving medical treatment in good faith on a patient in an emergency without the

patient's knowledge or prior agreement. However, the presumption that all patients consent to medical treatment when their wishes are not known must be rethought in the case of the severely ill and the dying. Many times medical professionals feel forced to continue invasive medical treatments on patients whose wishes cannot be inferred with certainty, even when the effectiveness of such treatments is poor and the burdens are high.[11]

The medical mandate to prolong life clearly has its place, especially in situations in which aggressive medical treatment is likely to lead to a healthy, happy existence for the patient. In the case of the dying patient, however, the value of the rescue credo must be critically evaluated. Patients unquestionably have the right to fight for life even when the odds are poor, but they should not be pressured to endure interventions that may prolong life while at the same time increasing physical or emotional suffering. Although some would criticize those patients who do not elect to undergo every procedure that might buy them another few days of life, Quill censures this harsh puritanical approach to fighting death that seems to pervade current medical thinking. "Going 'gentle into that good night' with one's dignity and sense of self intact," he argues, "is certainly as morally acceptable as raging 'against the dying of the light.'"[12]

Despite the fact that the rescue credo of modern medicine may still be prominent, physicians and others increasingly appreciate the value of confronting death openly and carefully evaluating the benefits and burdens of aggressive medical treatment. Many recognize Elizabeth Kübler-Ross as being among the first to break ground in this area with her 1969 book, *On Death and Dying*. Kübler-Ross espoused dealing with death and the dying patient sincerely and compassionately. Her candid perspective is reflected in her own description of the book:

It is not meant to be a text book on how to manage dying patients, nor is it intended as a complete study of the psychology of the dying. It is simply an account of a new and challenging opportunity to refocus on the patient as human being . . . so that we may learn more about the final stages of life with all its anxieties, fears, and hopes. I am simply telling the stories of my patients who shared their agonies, their expectations, and their frustrations with us. It is hoped that it will encourage others not to shy away from the "hopelessly" sick but to get closer to them, as they can help them much during their final hours. The few who can do this will also discover that it can be a mutually gratifying experience; they will learn much about the functioning of the human mind, the unique human aspects of our existence, and will emerge from the experience enriched and perhaps with fewer anxieties about their own finality.[13]

The Hospice Movement and Comfort Care

Kübler-Ross's views were not welcomed at first by other physicians at her hospital or in other hospitals, where it wasn't the corporate aspiration to be known as a great places to die. Parenthetically, just ten years later, as part of an effort to make use of every floor at the new University of Massachusetts Hospital, my colleagues and I were able to start a hospital-based hospice. Within two or three years, as the hospice movement caught on in America, that hospice was relocated into the community. It was patterned after the efforts of Cicely Saunders in Great Britain to provide peaceful, caring environments—without aggressive medical treatment—for patients facing death. Hospice care takes place in special facilities ("hospices") and, probably more often, in home care programs. A multidisciplinary team of providers, including physicians, nurses, social workers, volunteers, and clergy deliver hospice care, often in concert with a patient's family members. Hospice programs have proliferated in the past thirty years; the mid-1980s hospice care qualified for support under Medicare.

The heart of a hospice program has been called "palliative" or "comfort" care. Comfort care is a humane approach to the medical treatment of incurably ill patients that focuses on the patient's quality of life, personal desires, and symptom alleviation. Although comfort care is most commonly associated with hospices, it can be used in any clinical setting.

Unfortunately, comfort care is usually offered quite late—only after all possibly effective treatments have been exhausted and the patient is near death—if it is offered at all. It is usually presented with an apology, as if the physician had failed to help, rather than positively, as a legitimate and valuable approach. Comfort care is less frequently explored with patients whose quality of life is deteriorating and for whom acute medical treatments are increasingly arduous. Quill explains why: "For some physicians, the comfort care philosophy threatens deeply held traditional medical values. Many see their primary mission as fighting for life, and easing the passage to death has no place in that fight."[14]

Many of those who have studied death have observed that physicians sometimes even abandon dying patients for whom there are no more technological options. It seems likely that physicians remove themselves out of their discomfort with death and helplessness to stop it. Nuland relates this abandonment to his previously described concept of "The Riddle":

As long as there is any possibility of solving The Riddle, they [physicians] will keep at it, and sometimes it takes the intervention of a family or the patient himself to put an end to medical exercises in futility. When it becomes obvious, though, that there is no longer a Riddle on which to focus, many doctors lose the drive that sustained their enthusiasm.[15]

The problems of abandonment and neglect of comfort care options probably have some roots in the experience of undergraduate and postdoctoral medical training. Quill notes:

> In teaching hospitals, most patients are no longer seen by medical students or residents when the decision is made to treat them with comfort care. It is felt to be a waste of the trainee's valuable time when they are "not going to do anything." "Not doing anything" translates into not undertaking traditional, disease-oriented medical treatments; but by implication it devalues the many complex medical options still available to comfort the terminally ill. The clear message is given that caring for the dying has less importance than caring for those who will use the medical technology to fight for life.[16]

On the other hand, comfort care does not mean active euthanasia. As Pellegrino points out, compassion does not encompass assisted suicide, and I agree with his insistence on this point. It cannot on balance be healthy for patients to wonder whether their doctors might decide they have suffered enough and help them out of life as a matter of professional judgment. Those interested in the ethics of physician-assisted suicide should read Dr. Quill's arguments and criteria in favor of it in certain instances and Dr. Pellegrino's response presenting the ethical arguments against such physician behavior.[17, 18]

In the range of possible futures for people arriving in a major urban hospital without a living will or advance directive to guide the caregivers are the following: an expensive, possibly futile course of treatment extended for as long as payments are forthcoming; blindly aggressive care unwilling to admit defeat until death supervenes; or options aimed at reducing pain, discomfort, and human isolation.

Progress

A number of hospitals have recently endeavored to develop ethical and compassionate protocols for providing care to terminally ill patients. For example, Texas's Hermann Hospital has developed a Supportive Care Protocol through its Program on Humanities and Technology in Health Care, led by Stanley Reiser, Lawrence Tancredi, and Cheves Smyth. The protocol establishes clear guidelines for the implementation of decisions concerning supportive care for terminally ill patients. It recognizes specifically that

> patients and their families (or other surrogate decision makers) may make decisions about health care that include changing, limiting, declining, or discontinuing a particular treatment, whether life-sustaining or otherwise ... The hospital's philosophy is to promote and protect patient dignity in the face of impending death by instituting medically appropriate care. Comfort will be maintained at all times through the provisions of analgesics, hygienic care, and other appropriate medical and nursing care to all patients.

Protocols like these reflect the hospital and health care establishment's increased willingness to deal with issues concerning dying patients. Living wills, advance directives, and health care proxies, all of which give people greater power of self-determination, also represent positive steps toward our society's acceptance of death. Such tools also help build a better dialogue between the clinical professions and the patients they serve, on the issue of end-stage treatment.

Through its consistent activities during the 1980s, the Robert Wood Johnson Foundation has dramatically improved hospital culture regarding humane care for the terminally ill and their families. After those involved in the foundation's efforts concluded that doctors' behavior couldn't be altered, they inserted a nurse family communicator into the mix, but results did not immediately improve. Ultimately though, for reasons that are unclear, hospital environments and treatment of the terminally ill improved significantly. My interpretation is simply that the Robert Wood Johnson Foundation's dogged investment in educating health leaders, professionals, and patients finally succeeded.

Medical schools have also made some progress in their approach to teaching about death. Classes on death and dying are offered at many schools, utilizing the large body of literature that now exists on the subject. The idea that the study of death could benefit from an emphasis on its meaning for individuals and societies, instead of an emphasis on its physiological correlates, has received increasing support in the last three decades. Indeed, Dr. Pauline Chen, in her recent book *Final Exam*, offers an extraordinarily sensitive story of her own growth as a young physician and surgeon through her encounters with death and dying patients.[19] Her experience shows how far medical education has progressed since my first encounter with death in 1959 and how far society as a whole still has to go in this regard. She points out that as of a few years ago, 100 percent of medical schools reported having formal educational programs on death and dying.

What Can We Do?

Physicians and clinical caregivers in general need to better understand the social and psychological aspects of death—and perhaps even some of the unconventional approaches to care found to be therapeutic—so as to develop a more consistently humane approach to caring for the dying. In my view, these are matters for a lifetime of professional study in which the goal should be steady improvement. Good communication skills are an essential ingredient in understanding patients' end-stage wishes, be they for aggressive intervention or comfort care. Encouraging patients to complete advance directives is one way physicians can initiate discussion about death and dying with their patients. Perhaps most important, advance directives relieve the ambiguity that can make death and dying in a medical setting so ominous.

Physicians must also explore their own beliefs about death. Not only can this sort of self-reflection ease anxiety about death, it can help the physician to override any influence that his or her personal values may be having on treatment decisions that truly belong to the patient. Having contemplated their own beliefs about death, physicians are also better equipped to handle situations in which a patient's wish to die includes a request for assisted death. Physician-assisted death raises many difficult moral questions and involves a snarl of legal and professional complications.[20, 21]

My own experience with dying patients has pointed to a seemingly simple yet powerful strategy for dealing with death: loyalty to stand by the patient to ensure that everything appropriate is provided, including companionship and attention by the clinical caregivers, family, and friends. Often, just sitting by a patient's side is the best medicine of all—for both clinician and patient. The presence of someone who expresses a caring attitude, whether silently or with words, can significantly enhance a patient's well-being, irrespective of the degree of his or her illness. So too can such companionship benefit the clinician. In most cases, the clinician cannot and perhaps should not be physically present for long periods of time. However, in most cases it is important that clinicians check in regularly with those who are present and with the patient. Clinicians who decide that their presence and attention are no longer necessary or useful in the case of terminally ill patients with no further treatment options may be selling both themselves and their patients short.

The experienced clinician realizes that all decisions, both diagnostic and therapeutic, are provisional and subject to revision as time passes and circumstances change. With that realization comes the understanding that the foundation of competent continuing care is the clinician's commitment to stick with the patient, no matter what turn the course of illness takes. This is not always an easy prescription to follow. The ability to carry it out is an important indicator of professional and personal maturity, for both individuals and our enlarging care teams.

An often unspoken question is whether increasing clinical specializations, time constraints, and other bureaucratic or social obstacles get in the way of a personal approach. Clinicians may worry. What will others think? Am I wasting time? Is this an appropriate use of my time? How is this time counted or billed? In novels, movies, and TV series episodes, doctors commonly exit a scene saying, "There is nothing more I can do." Given that doctors are trained to heal, rescue, or aid recovery, not to be experts in assisting the dying, do doctors and other clinicians simply feel they are inadequately prepared or trained for this part of their job?

The answer is that it is the responsibility of every clinician, whether a primary care physician, hospitalist, or specialist, to do whatever is possible to arrange companionship, comfort care, and continuing personal attention, however brief, for dying patients and their families. Good doctors and nurses have learned to remember these things. The clinicians in charge at any given time should keep dying patients on their to-do lists. In the hospital setting, the doctor and nurse on their rounds should not pass the patient's door without stopping in, even if the family is present. If the deathbed is at home, a telephone call serves just as well.

I cannot end this discussion without emphasizing the potential richness of a personal experience with the dying, once there is a chance to reflect on it. My father was a heavy smoker, when that was more than socially acceptable. He was otherwise healthy when he collapsed in the bathroom, paralyzed from the waist down. He was quickly diagnosed with lung cancer with metastases to the lower spine, transecting his spinal cord. After some weeks of rehabilitation, he went home in a wheelchair. One night, my mother called to tell me that she had called the ambulance and they were going to the hospital. She gave him the telephone, apparently just as the ambulance arrived, and he said, "Rog, I think this is it!" I said I was on the next plane and would see him in the morning. When I arrived three thousand miles and twelve hours later, he was in coma and died within hours.

Seven years afterward, my mother, also an inveterate heavy smoker throughout her life, was in effect a pulmonary cripple in her eighties. She was cared for in a nearby nursing home and I was able to visit frequently. It was no surprise when I got a call that she seemed near death and that I should come quickly. I was there within half an hour, and as I entered the room I found her with a nun who seemed to be a specialist in these transitions. My mother looked up at me, smiled benevolently, and returned her attention to the nun. Her face seemed angelic—and instead of the tearful good-bye I had anticipated, it was clear she was busy with more important matters. I left the room and waited outside. When I returned, she had passed.

Reflecting on these two episodes from my own family history, I am reminded of the words of John J. McDermott, whom I have already mentioned as a distinguished American philosopher and a longtime friend. In an essay on the prospect of his own death, he asks, "How is it possible that a vicarious experience [i.e., of someone else's death] can have such a direct hold on our deepest feelings and our most intense of personal anticipations?"[22] He notes that the inevitability of death is so repressed in our society that the news that someone else is terminally ill seems devastating to those who will remain. He advises celebrating our lives in all their details, cherishing what we can of life while we have it, and summarizes the bottom-line conclusion of his essay by saying:

> At some point in our life, the sooner the better, we should confront the inevitability of our own death and absorb this awareness into the most active forefront of our consciousness. The message is clear and two-fold: avoid the temptation to invest in meaning which transcends our own experience of the life-cycle; and affirm the immanence of death as the gateway to an unrepressed life in which the moment sings its own song, in its own way, once and only once.[23]

For him, it is the celebration of the ordinary that can enable us to make our own way as truly human, and he observes that this need not involve belief in everlasting life.

Recently, as I was reflecting on what health professionals should be aware of as they attempt to support patients and families in our increasingly racially and culturally diverse population, the work of two modern intellectuals got on my radar. The ideas of Ernest Becker and his followers,[24] and some of those expressed by the brilliant and outspoken atheist biologist Richard Dawkins in his book *The God Delusion*,[25] should prove of value to caregivers who wish to serve patients as much as possible on their own terms, whatever they may be.

Both of these thinkers emphasize the centrality of death to our lives, even as we approach a vanishingly small and shrinking near-term future prior to an impending demise. Ernest Becker, a distinguished social scientist, theorizes that human behavior (constructive or destructive, good or evil) flows from our anxiety about our often subconscious but intense awareness of mortality. In his last book,

Escape from Evil,[26] as well as in earlier work on the philosophy of education, he points to ways in which we can tame our destructive anger and make it constructive. In thinking about my own days as a patient, I came to believe that I was happier in those moments when I could still focus, however briefly, on other people rather than myself. Certainly, if one makes it through a health crisis, such an approach can add value and happiness to whatever life remains.

Dawkins reminds us in *The God Delusion* that however many Americans believe in a hereafter and a personal god, a significant number of patients do not. He is such a passionate atheist that I wondered as I read along how he thought he might face his own death. His last chapter answers the question, celebrating atheist heroes like Bertrand Russell and Peter Medawar and dismissing religious consolation. Dawkins looks forward to dying happy that he had the extraordinary good fortune to have been a product of genetic pieces that came together, survived, and matured. And that he saw and understood more of the universe through science than he had ever dreamt possible. I understand that Dawkins wants no talk of religion at his time of dying, but to my mind his words of thankfulness and reverence for the marvels of the universe could have come from Teilhard de Chardin, the anthropologist priest who said he never felt closer to God than when he was doing science.

I hope these reflections about death and dying may be useful, at the right time, to caregivers and patients alike. In confronting our own or others' end of life challenges, it may be helpful to recall those who lost their lives while fulfilling a commitment to moral and ethical principles, religion, or country. In conclusion, let me suggest that every so often not only doctors, nurses, and patients, but also those leading our communities and businesses could benefit from reading the brief items below:

It came to me the other day:
Were I to die, no one would say,
"Oh, what a shame! So young, so full
Of promise—depths unplumbable!"
Instead, a shrug and tearless eyes
Will greet my overdue demise;
The wide response will be, I know,
"I thought he died a while ago."

For life's a shabby subterfuge,
And death is real, and dark, and huge.
The shock of it will register
Nowhere but where it will occur.

"Requiem," John Updike[27]

No runs, no hits, no errors . . . no serious errors!

"Nantucket Death Announcement,"
Alan Brown[28]

Part II

Elements for Successful Adaptation in the Twenty-first Century

Chapter 6

Unity in Diversity with Patients and Populations

Our nation's health care system has been justly criticized for costing too much and serving too few. Miraculous operations like organ transplants are commonplace in America's high-tech hospitals, yet millions go without basic medical care because they cannot afford it. The media report on widespread cholera in Africa or outbreaks of avian or swine flu,[1] yet preventable epidemics of dental caries and rampant gum infections, with their serious consequences for overall health, go undiagnosed and untreated in large numbers of American minority children. Although among developed countries the United States by far spends the most on health care, it has the highest infant mortality and shortest adult life spans. America's haves do not lag on these measures, but its burgeoning numbers of have-nots might as well be living in another country.

The roots of these ironic circumstances run deep. They illustrate a fundamental tension between our societal emphasis on individualism, enshrined as our right to "the pursuit of happiness" in the Declaration of Independence, and our responsibility for the common good, as stated in the Constitution's emphasis to "promote the general welfare." Balancing these goals has become a far more complicated undertaking than when our great national documents were written in the eighteenth century.

Many see this tension in the rift between two professions that play major roles in maintaining health: medicine and public health. Claims that the health care crisis can only be solved through the union of medicine and public health figure in reform proposals, curriculum debates in schools of medicine, nursing, public health, and plans for allocating federal research dollars. There are calls for primary care doctors to practice in community health centers, for physicians and other providers to counsel their patients about the link between behavior and disease, and for medicine to follow epidemiology's lead on preventable environmental risk factors and threats to health. That public health and medicine should partner in promoting and maintaining health seems eminently logical. Yet the rift between them began with the birth of public health as a distinct area of endeavor. In many respects that rift has never narrowed.

Public Health's Beginnings

Throughout history, epidemics of diseases like plague, cholera, and smallpox have evoked scattered public efforts to protect the health of population groups through isolation of the ill and quarantine of travelers.[2] These efforts occurred despite the fact that epidemic disease was often believed to be a sign of poor moral and spiritual condition. In the nineteenth century a surge of discoveries in bacteriology, identifying filth as both a cause and vehicle of transmission for disease, brought about "the great sanitary awakening."[3] Momentous discoveries in the latter half of the century by scientists like Robert Koch, whose now famous postulates revealed the link between microorganisms and certain diseases, transformed the way epidemics were understood and combated.[4]

The sanitary awakening, coupled with the birth and flourishing of medical microbiology, spurred an embrace of cleanliness and a dramatic shift in the way society thought about health. Illness was now regarded as an indicator of poor social and environmental conditions.[5] Perhaps most significant, these events also changed the way society thought about public responsibility for communal health.

As historian Elizabeth Fee notes, "Poverty and disease could no longer be treated simply as individual failings."[6] Public sewage drainage, waste disposal, and water purification systems were put into place, as were public hospitals, one of the most significant signs of public acceptance of responsibility for citizens' health. As a result of Louis Pasteur's work late in the nineteenth century, immunization also came into increasing use as a strategy for controlling, and even preventing, some diseases like smallpox. Together these circumstances—the growth of knowledge about sources of disease and strategies for controlling them and public acceptance of disease control as both feasible and obligatory—shaped the development of the field of public health.

Public Health, Medicine, and Professional Turf

Initially, medicine and public health became allies in the effort to maintain the health of communities. The two fields shared in their investment in epidemiology, the study of populations. The membership of professional epidemiological societies included many practicing clinicians.[7] Ironically, the paths of medicine and public health began to diverge just as advances in bacteriology produced increasing evidence that they ought to be merged. Not surprisingly, tension over professional turf was at the heart of the matter.

One of the pivotal events in the history of relations between the public health establishment and the practicing clinical community was the discovery that both the environment and people could be agents of disease. Although previously focused on environmental sanitation, public responsibility for health came to encompass individual health as well. This brought public health professionals into competition with physicians, in that control measures such as immunizations were carried out not in the environment but on individual patients, who were the purview of the private doctor.[8]

Medical sociologist Paul Starr relates a story about tuberculosis control efforts in the late nineteenth and early twentieth centuries, when tuberculosis notification by private doctors was made mandatory, that illustrates the tensions between medicine and public health. He writes in *The Social Transformation of American Medicine*:

> There was ordinarily no interference with patients under the care of private practitioners, and other consumptives were generally only visited by medical inspectors, who left circulars and gave advice about preventing the spread of infection. But fear of tuberculosis was widespread, and many people were anxious about any official report of its presence in their family; some life insurance policies were void if tuberculosis was the cause of death. Objecting that tuberculosis was not contagious, practitioners opposed compulsory reporting as an invasion of their relationships with patients and of patients' rights to confidentiality. The president of the New York County Medical Society told its membership in 1897 that by requiring notification and offering free treatment, the health department was "usurping the duties, rights, and privileges of the medical profession."[9]

A different sort of tension separating clinicians and public health professionals has been the growing tendency of the latter to function as assessors, evaluators, and critics of medical practice. An early clue to this tension can be gleaned from the tragic story of the great nineteenth-century Viennese obstetrician Ignaz Semmelweis, who discovered how to protect women from dying from puerperal sepsis after childbirth, only to have this discovery rejected by his colleagues in the medical community. Semmelweis observed lower mortality rates in a clinic staffed by midwives than in one staffed by doctors and medical students. He deduced that in the latter, clinicians were carrying infection from patient to patient and from autopsy to patient. Also, recognizing the similarity at autopsy between death from puerperal sepsis and death from wound infection, Semmelweis pointed to the efficacy of hand washing with lime before attending deliveries.

The medical community, however, was unwilling to accept the link between hand washing and infection (these events having taken place many years prior to the sanitary awakening). For his outspoken advocacy, Semmelweis was derided and effectively drummed out of the medical corps.[10] He died in an asylum, broken in spirit, while young women continued to die by the thousands thanks to the blindness and inflexibility of entrenched practitioners. Another way of explaining the opposition to Semmelweis's discovery is to return to recent neuroscience findings, discussed in chapter 2, which indicate that certainty is a feeling generated by the somewhat primitive midbrain and may not be easily affected by the rational dispositions of the cerebral cortex.

The increasing role of the "clinical evaluative sciences" exemplifies this tension as it persists today. The clinical evaluative sciences refer to the application of epidemiology, sociology, anthropology, and statistics to the assessment of health care. This research is by its very nature an activity outside the delivery of services. In many instances, what emerges is a tension between the active agent, the clinician, and the critic, the evaluative scientist or public health practitioner, with the latter telling the world about the inadequacy of the former. The stress of the situation is compounded when the active agent is a specialist who perceives him- or herself to be in the higher echelons of technical accomplishment. Such an agent tends to dismiss epidemiologic studies because they address the average level of competence—the collective success—and undervalue what the extraordinary surgeon or practitioner can achieve.

Political events have also kept medicine and public health at odds. Shortly after World War I, for example, when public health workers tended to support national health insurance, the relationship between medicine and public health soured further. Post–World War II federal initiatives in health care for the poor and elderly exacerbated already sensitive relations.[11] Organizational arrangements in education and service functions solidified the rift. Population-based science— epidemiology informed by and in concert with demography, anthropology, sociology, economics, and health statistics—developed in schools of public health separate from medical schools. Likewise, state and regional authorities established public health departments outside the personal health care system. Suspicion, tension, and isolation persist in many sectors, although relations between medicine and public health have improved in recent years. For example, the Association of Schools of Public Health and the Association of American Medical Colleges have developed and sustained increasing numbers of collaborative efforts over the past decade.

Philosophical Differences

Paul Starr's account of tuberculosis control efforts illustrates the friction between medicine and public health over professional turf, but it also touches on something that has emerged as perhaps the most dominant force behind the separation of the two fields: the fundamentally different scientific paradigms under which they operate and conceptualize their activities. Most physicians and medical school faculties operate under the Newtonian, reductionist, biomedical model, which emphasizes the understanding of disease and therapeutics at the molecular level. Doctors tend to focus on the molecular intervention that will bring about a particular effect in an individual patient. Public health practitioners, on the other hand, work with a variety of disciplines, especially epidemiology. Such professionals think about populations, demographic trends, and overall morbidity and mortality statistics. Medicine focuses on disease and its treatment; public health focuses on prevention. Medicine seeks to understand the pathogenesis of poor health; public health seeks strategies for the promotion of good health. Medicine aims to improve the health of individuals; public health aims to improve the conditions of life for all people in the community.

The struggle boils down to a patient-centered versus a population-based approach. Yet increasing evidence indicates that individual patients would benefit from being treated in the context of what is known about the populations to which they belong. The growing number of medical conditions known to have their origins in environmental, behavioral, and sociological factors has made this increasingly undeniable. In the past fifty years, mortality rates from infectious diseases have declined dramatically, whereas mortality rates from cancer, injuries, and chronic diseases of the cardiovascular system have increased dramatically. This means that the agent responsible for death and disability has shifted increasingly from the microorganism to the person and society. At least in developed countries, the list of most critical disease vectors no longer includes contaminated water supplies or insects. Instead, it features abundant but unhealthy diets that have escalated rates of diabetes and other metabolic and autoimmune illnesses; the automobile; environmental pollutants in and out of the food chain; and nicotine, alcohol, and other drugs.[12] This "new morbidity" has made the need for teamwork between public health and medicine especially urgent.[13]

Many experts say that public health gives inadequate attention to the biological sciences and thus hampers the ability of public health practitioners to understand the procedures, technologies, and treatments they are charged to evaluate. But a larger chorus of experts argues that the medical profession's insistence on maintaining an unnatural separation from public health has restricted the health benefits to individuals and communities that could accrue from health promotion and disease prevention activities. The medical profession is now striving to understand the faults of the medical approach and identify targets for change.

For most of the twentieth century, medical schools have predominantly focused on two areas: (1) concern with cellular and molecular disease processes (laboratory based) and (2) care of one patient at a time (clinical).[14] Although the value of what has been achieved in biomedical research laboratories has been tremendous—as evidenced by early medical miracles like antibiotics and more recent breakthroughs like gene therapy—there has been a serious imbalance in the two pursuits. The overarching gestalt of modern medicine has become associated with specialization, super specialization, and an explosion of interventions and technologies. This is, many observers believe, to the exclusion of other equally important considerations bearing on the patient's care and well-being. Critics argue that in its intense concentration on research and technology designed to unravel disease mechanisms in individual patients, medicine has become overly disease oriented, losing touch with the very people suffering from disease.

In an essay on the role of physicians in health promotion, physician Bob Lawrence points out the tendency for the awe-inspiring technologies of modern medicine to overshadow public health strategies, which are frequently less dramatic and glamorous. He writes:

In health promotion, we encounter issues of personal behavior, culture, values, and law. The triumphs of modern medicine are the results of experimentations and reductionism, of systematic attempts to remove all consideration of personal behavior, culture, and the like, to understand biologic systems.[15]

As Lawrence also notes, the more immediate feedback provided by successful treatment of symptomatic disease reinforces the physician's interest in pathology and therapeutics rather than in prevention or health promotion. Health promotion presents no "riddle" for physicians to solve: the emphasis is on health, a nonevent. Richard Pels and colleagues point out that health promotion involves "no dramatic surgical intervention, and the grateful patient is replaced by someone unlikely to credit, much less praise, the physician for improving the probability of a longer and better life."[16] Moreover, epidemiological research, by its nature and scope, can be slow in its returns, although the returns can be particularly powerful. In retrospect, we have been appallingly slow to recognize the serious disparities in health that epidemiological research reveals among our many racial, ethnic and socioeconomically diverse subpopulations.

Naturally, many people have looked to the training of physicians to understand how the rift between medicine and public health has endured. Clues are abundant. Most medical students load their premedical curriculum with the biological and chemical sciences, a pattern that continues into medical school, at least for the first two years. Lacking, and sometimes altogether missing, from medical curricula is formal exploration of the society in which students will diagnose and treat people when they graduate. Physician and medical sociologist Leon Eisenberg offers a possible explanation for the short shrift given to the social sciences:

There is widespread skepticism among physicians as to whether psychological and social factors are as "real" as biological ones. Classroom exercises will have convinced all of them of the power of biological reductionism. It is not only that so much more time is devoted to the natural as opposed to the "unnatural" sciences in medical education, but that the elegance of molecular biology is so much greater.[17]

The infrastructure of medical education may also be a barrier to the study of communities. Much of medical education takes place at the bedside of sick individuals receiving highly specialized care in hospitals, even though demographic and lifestyle shifts have greatly reduced our society's need for such care. Historically, outpatient service, the hospital's greatest link to the community, has been viewed as a charitable impulse, not as a site for medical education.[18] Positive steps have been taken in the reshaping of admissions criteria and in the blossoming of community-based preceptorships and departments of community medicine But it takes time to alter long-ingrained patterns of behavior.

Today, as always, physicians are trained to be problem solvers and to focus on the physical symptoms of the patient. Physicians typically are not trained to think in terms of prevention, health promotion, or social or psychological influences on health. In the words of one observer, physicians work in a "sickness industry," which may explain why they have been known to ignore things like child abuse, believing the issue is none of their business.[19] Whereas physicians frequently provide secondary or tertiary preventative services (e.g., blood-cholesterol-lowering drugs to prevent cardiovascular problems), the notion of primary prevention, that is, altering risk factors before they can begin to influence disease processes, is something most physicians still relegate to the domain of public health practitioners.[20]

Several studies report that physicians lack confidence in their ability to motivate behavioral change in their patients and believe they are poorly trained to practice preventive medicine.[21, 22] Confidence tends to increase with level of training; lack of confidence typically correlates with no effort to counsel patients and early cessation of counseling when working with poorly motivated patients.[23] Surveys have also documented that physicians frequently do not adhere to preventative practice recommendations because they perceive them as ambiguous or conflicting.[24] The literature can indeed be confounding, as anyone trying to discern whether butter or margarine will clog the arteries faster could attest. Part of the frustration here may lie with the poor coordination between health services and the evaluative sciences, which are still in large part sequestered in the domain of public health. Not least of the reasons that physicians may find it a challenge to assimilate new findings into their practices is the pace at which biomedical research moves forward.

Constraints of the practice setting can also hamper physicians' prevention and health promotion activities. Lack of support services and the time pressures of busy primary care practices can interfere with the delivery of prevention and health promotion services, even when these are recognized as important.[25] In addition, many practices simply do not have easy access to dieticians, smoking cessation groups, substance dependence counselors, and other referral services that can provide both support and education around health promotion interventions.[26]

Joining Forces

Given the huge number of preventable deaths that occur each year due to the consumption of nicotine, alcohol, and other substances, among other risky behaviors, the great challenge to physicians is to devote more attention to helping patients adopt healthy habits. The great challenge for patients is to take greater responsibility for their own health promotion and disease prevention. This is where the patient's role as figurative chair of the board of a personal health care company is most obviously important.

Rising numbers of injuries, chronic diseases, and sexually transmitted diseases send a loud, clear signal of the need for health care providers to stress disease prevention and health promotion. Increases in obesity and diabetes; disease traced to diets with excessive amounts of fat, salt, and sugars; deafness from noise pollution; brain tumors and who knows what else from excessive exposure to handheld electronic devices and cell phones; and cell phone–associated auto, train, plane, and bus accidents all illustrate how public health and medicine need each other. Separately, the contributions of each field to improving the nation's health have been profound. Together, through coordination of each field's unique strengths, they can achieve even more.

Nurses are the health professionals who could best work with patients through ambulatory health facilities and with schools, churches, and local governments to provide public information of the highest quality. The federal government could support an expanded role for nurses in this regard, as part of its clear responsibility for public education in environmental and toxicological matters and other health related and prevention services.

Although we probably cannot expect to train enough physicians to meet the demand in this area, reshaping the medical school curriculum is an important starting point in bringing medicine and public health closer together. Even if the vast majority of physicians continue to devote themselves to private practice, they need knowledge of statistics and epidemiological concepts in order to treat their patients effectively and efficiently. Equally important, knowledge of population-based approaches facilitates understanding of other vital elements that affect the natural history and management of illness. As outlined in the Health of the Public, a medical education reform initiative of the Pew Charitable Trusts and the Rockefeller Foundation, instruction in diagnosis, treatment, and prevention must address not only the individual patient but also the community. This is where the determinants of health and the factors influencing the severity of illness resulting from disease can be measured and modified.[27] A number of forward-thinking medical schools were early adopters and assimilated these considerations in their students' educational experience. By now, most schools emulate this example.

If training of physicians and other health care professionals must more fully integrate the principles of community-based comprehensive care, public health curricula must also include the principles of biology, biomedicine, and reductionist, biomolecular interventions. This is especially true, given the prospect that advances in genetic medicine will make it possible to predict disease risks from a drop of blood at birth. Future physicians will likely practice preventive genetics, treating healthy people before they get sick. From a pedagogical point of view, more effective interprofessional teaching and learning should thus serve to bring public health and medicine together.

Forty years ago, the concept of the academic health center took root with the founding of the Association of Academic Health Centers. Its membership comprises health-sciences universities and health-professional schools associated with the university clinics; and teaching hospitals within the framework of a parent university. Slowly but surely, entrenched professional fiefdoms are giving way to true teamwork and interprofessional collaboration. Nursing, dental, medical, and other health-related professions students are cross-pollinating in schools of public health, yielding more professionals educated both clinically and in public health. Over the past twenty years, the ranks of college and university presidents and chancellors have consequently come to include many educated in the health sciences. Prior to that such a professional background was highly uncommon.

As students choose among professional schools, they should include among their criteria the degree to which a school has forged links between its profession and other health professions on the one hand, and between individual patient care and population health on the other hand. Clearly, it is important for medicine to maintain the unique strengths of the medical approach. But the need for medical schools to be at the frontiers of innovation in technical and molecular medicine must not outweigh their obligation to shape their students and their services to meet the needs of the community. The same general statement could be made about dental, nursing, and other health professional schools, where many educators have been ahead of their medical school colleagues in this regard. Likewise, public health schools should maintain their unique strengths in epidemiology, environmental health, health promotion, and disease prevention, while better integrating the basic principles and some of the more technical elements of biomedicine. These would include the impacts of hard scientific advances (e.g., genetics, nanotechnology, and toxicology) on the health of the population at large.

I gained a deeper understanding of the medicine–public health divide, and how they can work together, when in 1978 I went to the University of Texas (UT) Health Science Center at Houston as its second president. There I came into contact with Dr. Ruell Stallones, a physician and public health academic. He was the founding dean of the UT School of Public Health (the first school of public health between the Mississippi River and the Pacific Coast), one of the major component institutions of the UT Health Science Center, along with schools of medicine and nursing. Dr. Stallones and his colleagues had admitted their first public health students in 1969, three years before the Texas legislature established the UT Health Science Center. As a staunch advocate for the public health paradigm, Dr. Stallones looked upon any president of the UT Health Science Center with guarded enthusiasm at best, especially one like me, whose previous post was dean of a medical school.

He wasted no time in sharing his view that because twentieth-century advances in health status tracked much more closely with certain improvements—in sanitation, nutrition, air and water quality, and economic and educational status—than with biomedical breakthroughs (like the discovery of antibiotics) the United States should be spending all its health research dollars on population-based studies. Instead it was devoting most of them to disease-specific biomedical investigations. On a cost-benefit basis there could not be one iota of doubt, he said, that epidemiology left biochemistry in the dust.

The argument compelled attention on its merits and on account of Dr. Stallones's impassioned eloquence. But the ledger was not blank on the other side. I in turn sought to persuade him of the potential for medicine and public health disciplines to achieve more through cooperation and collaboration than competition. In particular, I wanted him and his colleagues in public health not to keep their distance from biomedicine and its specialty- and technology-oriented physicians, whose decisions generate 70 percent of health care costs. By engaging with them, they could help these physicians make cost-effective decisions, freeing up money for increased and better health care for more Americans. Likewise, I wanted those in public health to learn more about biomedicine's fast-developing capabilities, so they could help the public derive the full benefit of those advances.

In the following years, Dr. Stallones and I worked together to further these aims at the UT Health Science Center and beyond. As a result, I think it is safe to say that the faculties and students of the schools of medicine and public health gained a better mutual understanding of their respective disciplines than many of their counterparts elsewhere. I was very sad when cancer cut short Dr. Stallones's exceptional contributions to the UT Health Science Center and the field of public health. Under his leadership, the UT School of Public Health had moved up many places to become number six, in research dollars generated, out of what were then twenty-six public health schools in the country. In the early 1990s, the educational and research culture he did so much to define had advanced to number three out of a larger number of schools, and it continues to be one of the country's leading public health schools. He features in two of my most cherished memories of my ten years in Houston. The first is his giving me a wonderful gold-threaded representation of the University of Texas symbol, signifying that I had at last passed his test of loyalty to my new university and state. The other is his spontaneous smile when he awoke briefly and recognized me visiting him with his wife at his deathbed.

Perhaps the most important breakthrough encouraging greater collaboration between medicine and public health has been the documentation of preventable deaths in hospitalized patients. As a result, there have been subsequent systematic approaches to improved safety and barrier-free communication across the industry over the past decade. Population-oriented public health professionals should also examine a phenomenon that I think of as the epidemiology of hope. I call it epidemiology because it is a population-based phenomenon. Paradoxically, it also gets to the heart of the patient-centered medical model.

An Epidemiology of Hope

With health care dollars tight, a more population-based approach to health care has a certain appeal. In some arenas, efforts have even been made to rank health interventions according to their public health impact and the "bang for the buck" they provide for a population. Plans have been considered to exclude from coverage expensive procedures that benefit only a small number of people. Prevention and health promotion activities have loomed large in every health care reform plan, because most of the time the costs of these activities are reasonable and their benefits real. It is certainly important to understand which interventions work well. It is also past time to curb inflation in health care costs driven by overutilization of high-tech treatments.

But there is something about the shift in orientation to a wholly population-based approach that feels strangely uncomfortable. The necessity of reforming the nation's health care system to better meet the needs of our population has become distressingly obvious. Yet we have not been able to reduce coverage for certain medical interventions—those either not proven effective or that are more costly than alternate, equally effective measures—and invest more of our scarce health care dollars in health promotion and disease prevention. I believe our reluctance has a lot to do with an epidemiology of hope, a typically American phenomenon.

By this I refer to the fact that every state in the nation has one or more major medical centers where the latest technologies and the most proficient specialists stand ready to treat serious illness or trauma. The high-tech medicine of our most advanced hospitals not only provides an extraordinary array of interventions for current patients, but also provides hope for all potential patients. This population-based hope, buttressed by laws requiring hospitals to treat everyone who has a dire emergency, allows us to believe that if something dreadful befalls us or a loved one, a dramatic intervention might provide a typically American new beginning.[28]

One such intervention has stayed with me since I witnessed it in the fall of 1956, two months after I entered medical school. Three other medical students and I eagerly accepted an invitation to observe what was then a revolutionary procedure, the open heart repair of complex, multifaceted heart defects—and in a newborn infant girl, a so-called blue baby!

In a room directly above the operating room, my fellow students and I sat down at a circular glass table. Across from us sat three visiting physicians, speaking what turned out to be Russian. The glass table allowed us all to see every movement of the surgical team at work below, led by Dr. Robert Gross, the pioneering innovator of this operation on blue babies, who would otherwise die an early death from cardiorespiratory failure.

It wasn't long before we saw technicians place a long narrow machine with vertical discs next to the operating table. This was the newly developed heart-lung pump oxygenator, through which the baby girl's blood would flow while Dr. Gross and his team tried to repair her multiple heart defects.

A surgical nurse carried in the baby girl, deep cyanotic blue from head to toe because her heart could not give her blood enough oxygen, and placed her on the operating table. The baby's circulatory system was connected to the heart-lung pump oxygenerator, and her blood became ever more red as it passed through the machine's oxygen-bathed discs and returned to her body. Within seconds, her skin changed from deep blue to the healthy pink of a normal infant.

In a surprisingly short period of time, the surgical team finished working on her heart and prepared to disconnect her circulatory system from the machine. The tension built as the team completed the last steps of the procedure. Now it was all up to the baby's lungs and her surgically repaired heart. I held my breath, then found myself cheering along with everyone else at the glass table and in the operating room, as the baby remained pink and rosy, heart pumping oxygen from lungs to blood normally for the first time in her brief, but now potentially long and promise-filled life.

The other students and I were ecstatic over this technological miracle and remained so. I felt extraordinarily lucky to be joining a profession that could work such wonders. The Russian doctors' initial enthusiasm quickly subsided, however. Through their interpreter, they congratulated Dr. Gross and his colleagues on a technological tour de force, but said that in Russia they simply preferred to have another baby. Rather than callousness, this statement probably expressed our three visitors' frustration at their comparative lack of such resources. It was, after all, the height of the Cold War, when none of them could be sure what the others might report to the KGB later. It was a dangerous thing in those days for a Russian to express too much admiration for anything American.

Forty years later, after the dissolution of the Soviet Union, I was a member of an American group visiting a children's hospital in the former Soviet Socialist Republic of Kazakhstan. Walking through the pediatric intensive care unit (ICU) with its Kazakhstani director, who was clearly proud of the unit and the entire hospital, I saw a blue baby in obvious cardiorespiratory distress and asked to go over to the infant. The ICU director's demeanor instantly changed, and he seemed near tears as we discussed the child's hopeless situation. Remarking that in America such babies underwent successful heart repairs every day, he said with great emotion, "We are all so without hope! It affects us all!"

It is not only in America that blue babies commonly undergo heart repair surgery these days; it also happens in other highly developed countries. But it is undoubtedly an especially American trait to want the capacity to test the limits of new technology and receive, or in the case of many physicians, provide another chance at a full life. The epidemiology of hope reflects our nation's embrace of individualism and our belief in the rights to life, liberty, and the pursuit of happiness as stated in our Declaration of Independence. The psychological value of this hope is well recognized by the military, which expends millions of dollars on elaborate systems of transportation and graded health care installations to assure its fighting cadres that if they are injured, everything will be done to save them. Public health–oriented interventions have also played on this characteristically

American, individualist hope for a second chance. Recall the slogan of the seat-belt campaign: "The life you save may be your own."[29]

With our current economic stress, hope of health for all motivates proposals to extend basic health care insurance to the 50 million uninsured Americans and to pay serious attention to the huge disparities in health care borne by various U.S. subpopulations.[30, 31, 32]

The American people watch with interest and pride as medicine rescues people from the brink of death.[33] The most awesome medical miracles occur in hospitals, yet three factors—their traditionally high-tech approach, their steep, administrative costs, and the movement of health care toward a more population-based, cost-conscious system—raise questions about how many such expensive high-tech institutions we need. Herein the epidemiology of hope comes into play, muddling the inquiry. Citizens may understand that their city has too many empty hospital beds, but still find themselves reluctant to support the closing of the nearest hospital, their emergency safety net. What if their loved one is in an auto accident or experiences a massive heart attack? Minutes could mean the difference between life and death.

We as a country will not easily yield these institutions to the budget ax. In all likelihood we will maintain our hospitals, which will increasingly become large intensive care units, dedicated to bringing people back from the brink. Hopefully, we will also economize and become much more prudent buyers of such care. Good health for our whole population will undoubtedly require greater investments in environmental and toxicological research and preventive health practices.[34, 35]

Once again, we shall all continue to need professional good judgment to balance the resources allocated between curative and preventive care. To have that balance among our health providers, we need it in our educational experiences. Although it is true that organized medicine and the public health establishment have frequently been at odds, it is important to realize that serious, responsible, and respected professional leaders are working hard to bridge the gap. Many are doing this by seeking training in medicine and public health and several, more recently, by experimenting with new kinds of educational venues and strategies. Even though I believe the "official" gap will disappear shortly, it will be up to the younger generation of caregivers to integrate the two intellectual paradigms, so that in the mind of each health care professional prevention and curing are seen as components of a continuum rather than as competitors.

The growing body of research on the environment's impact on public health heralds a vast new field of medical and health care expertise. This field will be important to both individual caregivers' practice habits and the agendas of health professional associations and advocacy groups. We will need a new workforce of environment- and population-based health information specialists, drawn most likely from the ranks of nurses, pharmacists, and physician-assistants. Doctors and dentists who specialize in this area will be in short supply, given that they take almost a decade to educate. But the growing trend toward a medical home, or more properly a health home—an entity that coordinates care, safeguards medical records, and enables patients to take charge of their own health care—should provide the opportunity for people and their caregiving teams to have access to the best and most reliable expert information.

Chapter 7

On Serving and Collaborating

Those considering becoming doctors, nurses, dentists, or other health care professionals should ask themselves, "Why do I want to do that?"

There are undoubtedly many appropriate motivations for a health care career. Having a range of values and interests driving the members of the health professions is a positive for both patients and the public. The health care workforce requires so many people, with such a wide variety of talents and skills, that it needs to attract all the appropriately talented people it can. But as far as possible, such people should carefully sort out their motivations. Unhappy clinicians will obviously be more likely to make patients unhappy with their care and reduce the quality of the health outcome.

For prospective physicians, choices among specialties like family medicine, pediatrics, internal medicine, and psychiatry or more technologically oriented specialties like radiology, pathology, and laboratory medicine generally cannot be made before medical school. Each area may attract people with different strengths in science and technique compared to interpersonal relationships. In certain areas of specialization, scientific skills should quite properly dominate interpersonal skills, because the care the specialist delivers is largely the technologic intervention, such as the laser treatment, the imaging scan, or the genetic manipulation.

Guido Majno, a world-renowned pathologist and biomedical scientist, has for many decades maintained a parallel scholarly interest in the history of medicine. A favorite teacher of mine in medical school, he was also chairman of the pathology department at the University of Massachusetts Medical School when I joined its faculty and administration in 1976. He has written authoritatively of the capacities of ancient healers, including the premodern fathers of Western scientific medicine. Majno contrasts their efforts to those of modern physicians:

> When scientific medicine began to perform its healing miracles (only fifty or sixty years ago), there was a marvelous opportunity. Ancient medicine had discovered the secret of helping souls. Now it was possible to help bodies as well, thanks to tons of knowledge, chemicals and machines.
>
> It did not quite work out that way. The new generation of scientific healers was carried away by the physical problems, in fact by anything that could be measured. Spiritual concerns are hard to measure. It was assumed that if the body is healed the rest would somehow follow.
>
> Before long the public began to realize that something was missing. We are now in the midst of a rising anti-medical tide, while scores of supposedly "holistic" would-be do-gooders move in to fill the vacuum. At the latest count, there are seventy alternative forms of medicine. They certainly have the secret cure—time—and they offer enough hope and smiles to heal eighty-five percent of all patients.

Majno suggests that it may be wrong to blame the problem on the teaching in medical schools:

The old ways are hard to teach; nobody yet has found a way to teach the human approach. Altschule [Dr. Marc Altschule was one of the most respected clinicians at Harvard Medical School during the mid and late twentieth century] has said, with characteristic irony, that "it cannot be taught—although it can be learned."[1]

Later, Majno seeks a remedy:

The message of history, as I have tried to decipher it, is that scientific therapy has eroded the human care which has always been a key part of the healing process. Young medical students, brought up in the system, may find it difficult or impossible to fight the trend. Maybe so, but there is hope. Awareness of the problem is a first step toward solving it ... It may be impossible to stretch minutes into hours, but the quality of those minutes can certainly be improved.[2]

Majno believes that by turning to the lessons of past masters of Western medicine and other forms of healing, physicians can learn how to use the precious and diminished time available to them to convey their human concern and their attentiveness to the patient's suffering. Through the marriage of humanity with the ever-burgeoning scientific arsenal of interventions, he argues, medicine can reverse the current antimedical trend and develop a corps of the most powerful healers the world has ever known.

The prospective physician must find an individual balance between the desire to provide direct human service and the need to master a wide variety of sciences and technologies. Mastering the medical sciences and keeping abreast of relevant developments throughout a professional lifetime require an intrinsic interest in and ability with the sciences. Without scientific knowledge and technical competence, all the good will in the world can only provide the patient with less than optimal care. Alternatively, high technical competence without the people skills to build trust and confidence is also far less than the optimal state for patients. The same alternatives apply in different degrees to those contemplating entering any of the health professions.

In the end, perhaps only the individual really understands her or his own motives. Certainly, only the individual can recognize the continuing ambiguity of her or his own motives on each new day of professional service. I hope my comments will raise some issues that may be useful for people contemplating a life in the so-called helping professions. Further, I hope patients will find these ideas helpful as they assess their choices among caregivers and health care organizations.

Service as an Idea

An old aphorism declares that there are two kinds of people in the world: those who use other people and those who serve other people. I have always felt uneasy with that particular oversimplification. My discomfort is abated if I can add a third category to which I believe I, and most other people, belong: those who sometimes use other people and sometimes serve them. Implicit in this third category is subclassification, separating those who wish they could serve others more of the time from those who wish they could use others more often and more effectively. Honest self-examination in relation to these categories may help guide those interested in one of the human service careers.

I have always felt that serious caregivers should see service as akin to a secular sacrament. Working in health care should transcend benevolent self-interest and the drive to please. Service can be very good business, but it is also something more fundamental than that for both the giver and the recipient of care. Gabriel Marcel, the great twentieth-century philosopher, mourns the debasement of the concept of service in the modern, bureaucratic, egalitarian state. He sees the giving of service to other human beings as the most fundamental human activity. What troubles Marcel about our increasingly bureaucratic society is not the drive for equality. It his perception that the typical citizen feels that he or she owes another individual only whatever the contract or the law or the mores of the society require—that much and no more.[3] It is instructive to think of his arguments, made many decades ago, in the context of some of the modern systems of health care with their heavy institutional overlay of values and procedures that govern the provision of service.

The physician-psychiatrist-social critic Robert Coles has written a book, *The Call of Service: A Witness to Idealism*, in which he relates several stories about people he has known and observed to have a unique commitment to giving service. When writing about his parents, he makes an important distinction between their different approaches to serving other people and the greater good. Coles describes his mother as a deeply religious person who explicitly connected her daily activities, her philosophy of living, and her religion. He describes his father, on the other hand, as someone who dedicated himself to serving others later in life and seldom articulated his reasons for doing so, being both more pragmatic ("Just do it!") and somewhat circumspect about what he might find if he probed his deepest motives. For Coles, both approaches to service are equally valid and meaningful.[4]

I had the pleasure of introducing Robert Coles at a noon lecture he gave at the UT Health Science Center. After I announced that the lecture would have to end at 1:00 p.m. on the dot because the next class would be there promptly, he went to the lectern without notes or slides, made eye contact with what seemed everyone in the room, and spun the fascinating story of the first black children who were brave enough to go to a previously all-white school. Probably three hundred students sat in rapt attention until exactly 12:59 p.m., when he wrapped up his talk without a hitch, a stammer, or a pause and left us all thinking about living up to the example set by those little kids. That may have been the best talk I have ever heard—and I have heard lots.

In *The Call of Service*, Coles relates an encounter with Thomas Merton and attempts to analyze the nature of the healing impact the contemplative monk and writer had on him and many others. According to Coles' analysis, Merton's power as a healer arose from the fact that he had known and continued to know personal suffering. Merton was able to ease others' burdens in the context of their knowledge that he shared personally in suffering. Of course, all of us have our burdens; Merton's gift came from being able to transmit both a sense of his own encounters with difficulties and a nonjudgmental acceptance of other people, whatever their difficulties. Coles writes:

Dorothy Day and Daniel Berrigan and Walker Percy and so many others sought Merton out. I especially remember Dorothy Day's remarks about him; "He had known much pain, and he knew how to lift pain from others." She was content to state those two aspects of Merton without connecting the one to the other in what people like me call a psychodynamic way. Nevertheless, she knew that an essential and important part of Merton's life was his passionate desire to minister unto others, to hear from them, learn of their tensions and turmoil, and tell them of his, too. Once Dorothy Day said this about Merton as we talked of his voluminous writing: "He cured with words—all the time he did! I know! I can remember those letters, the good medicine they were to me. And I always knew that with Merton it was the doctor healing himself as well as the rest of us who were his patients."[5]

Tensions between the Service Ethic
and the Ethos of
Scientific Clinical Practice

The best recent articulation of the divergent pulls of patient care and the science of medicine is surgeon Sherwin Nuland's *How We Die*. I've already mentioned Dr. Nuland's description of physicians' love for solving "The Riddle"—finding out in molecular terms the exact cause of every serious disease or symptom complex and doing something scientifically valid to address the problem.[6] This drive to solve The Riddle often brings the physician into direct conflict with the best interests of some patients, for whom the answer to The Riddle may be of no concern because they are in the process of dying and would like help with that, rather than high-cost technological hindrances to a peaceful passing.

Biomedical scientists compete with each other in solving riddles to an extent that I sometimes find troubling. There is an element of seeking the brass ring, of being the first to the intellectual moon, of receiving the recognition of the Nobel Prize or the financial rewards for discovering a fantastically useful genetic tool. More uniformly perhaps, the scientist is driven by the fun of the pursuit and by the challenge of the intellectual problem, rather than by a desire to serve suffering humanity.

Tracy Thompson, a writer whose life was dramatically altered for the better by the drug Prozac, interviewed its three creators to understand why they did it and what they felt upon reaching their goal. Thompson asked scientist Bryan Molloy, "How does it make you feel to know that what you have done has helped people—to know that this molecule that you invented has allowed me to live my life in a way I never thought possible?"

Molloy said, "This puts me in a somewhat embarrassing position . . . The company puts itself in the position of saying it is here to help people, and I'm here saying I didn't do it for that. I just wanted to do it for the intellectual high. It looked like scientific fun."[7]

Compare Molloy's motivation with what must have been at the root of Edward L. Trudeau's efforts. He was the famous physician and clinical investigator who in 1882 established the first sanatorium for tuberculosis patients, in the Adirondack Mountains of New York. Trudeau had contracted tuberculosis in 1873, when this often lethal malady was believed to be either inherited or caused by a perverted moral character; it was not thought to be infectious in origin. In 1887, he conducted a starkly simple and elegant experiment whose results convinced him and many others of the therapeutic benefits of fresh air, good nutrition, and ample rest, an approach which for half a century remained the most effective treatment for tuberculosis.

The experiment involved fifteen rabbits, divided equally into three treatment groups. Five rabbits were injected with *Tubercle bacilli*; they were then placed on an island (with no other rabbits) on which they could forage comfortably. One of these rabbits died of the disease; the other four recovered completely after fibrosis of the initial lesion. The five rabbits in the second group were also injected with *Tubercle bacilli*, but were kept in a limiting cage in a dark cellar, with minimal nutrition. All five died of tuberculosis. The last five rabbits were not injected with *Tubercle bacilli*, but they were put in the dark cellar with the same poor food as the second five. None of the last five rabbits died, although all lost weight on the regimen. Trudeau was doubtless self-interested in some respects, since he wanted to cure a disease he'd had, but he began his experiment after he recovered and no longer needed a cure for himself. That seems to put his motivation in a different category than the quest for honor, fortune, or intellectual achievement, although he achieved some if not all three.

Basic biomedical scientists, so-called pure scientists, may work at the frontiers of unexplored areas for years. During those years they are more likely to face disappointment than success in taking the next step forward. Furthermore, even successful work may not quickly, or even in their lifetimes, lead to diagnostic, therapeutic, or preventative interventions. Today's basic biomedical scientists sow the seeds of hope for tomorrow's health care. As an aside, this group of people provides the teachers for the basic science courses taken by aspiring health professionals, and the way medical school teachers treat students very much influences the way those students treat patients.

For Lewis Thomas, the physician-scientist turned writer and popular philosopher, the greatest motivation was the satisfaction of being useful to others. In an interview from his deathbed, published in the *New York Times* on November 21, 1993, by Roger Rosenblatt, Thomas said, "If we paid more attention to this biologic attribute, we'd get a satisfaction that cannot be attained from goods or knowledge. If you can contemplate the times when you've been useful, even indispensable, to other people, the review of our lives would begin to have effects on the younger generations ... plain usefulness."

So Lewis Thomas comes together in this regard with Thomas Merton, Gabriel Marcel, and Robert Coles. Bryan Molloy's honest answer shows us that "one size does not fit all" and reminds us that with people as with trees, "by their fruits you shall know them."

A Personal View of Service and Physicianhood

My understanding of my own motivation for working in the helping professions became clear to me a few years ago, during an interaction with my barber at the time. Diego was a naturalized citizen who combined great common sense and considerable cynicism about the world with a basic instinct that he should stay as far away from doctors and medicine as possible. During one of my haircuts, he commented that his right foot had just begun hurting, but he was sure the pain would go away soon. He didn't want to talk about any medicines.

At my next haircut two weeks later, Diego was obviously still in considerable pain. He volunteered that he was thinking about giving up active barbering and running his business from his desk. He had not seen a doctor, had no intention of doing so, and had taken no medications. It wasn't difficult for me to examine his foot and determine that he most likely was suffering from tendinitis. I suggested that he might get tremendous relief from some over-the-counter medicine and sitting down periodically. His response made it clear that the best way for me to achieve possible compliance from this nonpatient was to walk two blocks to the nearest pharmacy, buy the medicine, and bring it back to him. This I did, and noted his genuine surprise when I gave it to him.

I stopped in again the next morning on my way to work to see how he was. He reported no pain and registered renewed surprise that a doctor was doing all this at no charge to him. During the subsequent two years of my contacts with him, he remained pain free and had actually taken some precautions to protect against a recurrence. He felt he had been cured at least temporarily and was obviously much happier. It made me a lot happier to have made some correct guesses about how to help him get relief from his pain.

I realized, after feeling my satisfaction over his being pain free for the first time in a few weeks, that I was in fact a physician. I was impressed that my sense of satisfaction at this simple and routine intervention in a very commonplace disorder was every bit as great as it had been during those rare moments when I deciphered a complex medical problem, thereby solving a therapeutic riddle. Even though Diego's relief may have been psychological or pure chance, totally unrelated to any direct impact from the medicine, he felt better. I believe that for many other clinicians besides myself, it doesn't matter how simple or demanding the intervention required to solve the patient's problem may be; what matters most is that the patient feels better and the problem is solved.

My conclusion from all this is that caregiving health professionals are likely to be happiest in their work if helping others gives them real satisfaction. Do you like to hold a door open for another to pass through, or do you prefer that another holds the door open for you? Would you like to develop a healing presence as described by Coles in his essay on Merton, or would you prefer recommending an exercise or a pill and moving on to the next case? Although most tangible indices of service orientation are different for each person, these simple questions point to the importance of honest and careful self-reflection in selecting a career in which you can work both effectively and happily.

If you enjoy helping others—and if you are interested enough in science to keep learning in order to improve your scientifically based competencies—then in my view you are a candidate to become a twenty-first century healer and a member of the most powerful corps of healers the world has ever known. To do it best, young entrants must want to understand even those technologies at the edge of modern medical science, at least in a basic way, and to maintain that leading edge of knowledge throughout a professional lifetime. They must also rediscover the ancient verities of humaneness, civility, and caring described by Majno and work equally hard at becoming proficient and effective in the human relations arena.

What should you as a patient look for in a physician? Obviously, competence is the most important and obvious quality to seek, and no doubt the hardest to assess quickly. On a personal basis, it is revealing whether the doctor in question listens more than talks. A friend of mine in Texas, a surgeon named Red Duke, had an extraordinary bedside manner in that he looked with intense interest at anyone he was talking to, something his patients all responded to very positively. A few weeks after meeting him, I learned that he had been in an army armored division and was quite deaf from the big guns. When I realized that his bedside manner was partly attributable to his need to read lips and facial expressions (beneath that was his genuine concern for the patient's health), I learned something about making sure to look at patients while talking with them.

A negative attribute to watch for is the "gotta go" syndrome, which afflicts many busy people, including most doctors. But the best doctors don't give that impression all or most of the time. This is why sitting down even for two minutes can yield a more productive exchange. So my advice is, seek those who listen intently, like the hard of hearing Dr. Duke, and avoid those with the perpetual "gotta go" manner.

Collaboration in Service

People entering the clinical health professions today face a new challenge, or at least an old challenge with new and expanding dimensions. By this I refer to the expanding number of professionals on the health care delivery team and the increasing complexity of the health care delivery system. These developments have led to a variety of different teams often interacting with a single patient. It is no longer patient and doctor. It is patient and scores of members of the various health care teams brought to bear on his or her problems, within the context of the entire population and its overall health status. An individual caregiver's dedication to serve the patient is often no longer sufficient to achieve the desired outcome. Caregivers, institutions, and organizations must now learn to communicate and collaborate across professions in patients' interests.

Two noteworthy collaborative movements have illustrated how we can come together in complex situations to improve health care. The first, the Picker-Commonwealth Patient-Centered Care Program, resulted when the James Picker Foundation transferred its assets to the Commonwealth Fund, which then used those assets to make grants totaling nearly $10 million from 1987 to 1995. The grants funded interrelated programs to enhance communication between patients and their health care providers, especially by giving voice to the patients and coaching providers to listen better. The programs significantly improved health care outcomes for the patients involved, adding enormous impetus to the patient-centered concept and demonstrating the value of making the patient a de facto player on the health care team.[8] The fruits of this investment are still being reaped.

The second movement is more recent, more restricted in scope and focus, but even more compelling in showing how better teamwork can save thousands of lives lost every year through preventable medical errors and oversights. In *Why Hospitals Should Fly*, John Nance, a highly respected pilot and flight safety professional, calls for "barrier-free communication" within the health care team. His point of departure is the evidence he presents on flight safety in the airline industry, describing in convincing detail how everyone involved in an airplane's journey must be able to communicate immediately about safety-related matters without concern for authority or seniority.[9]

The stakes for patient safety are so high, the evidence delineating the scope and nature of the problem so convincing, and the proposed solutions so successful and promising, that every patient and health professional should learn what Nance has to teach about developing "interprofessional collegial health care teams." Barrier-free communication, which means more listening than talking and more humility than prideful self-interest, upends the traditional chains of command and authority in the health care system. To serve patients best and keep them safe, health professionals have to listen to all members of the team, not least of all the patients themselves. Nance's cogent analysis joins earlier, ongoing efforts to promote better health care teamwork, like the noteworthy achievements of the Kaiser Foundation Health Plan, described by former Kaiser CEO

David Lawrence in *From Chaos to Care: The Promise of Team-Based Medicine.*[10]

The goals of the movements for patient-centered care and better health care teamwork have not been fully achieved, but progress has been substantial. Institutional values have positive and negative impacts on individual values and behaviors. As such, the interplay between individual and organizational ethics will become increasingly important to the processes and outcomes of our health care delivery. Service-oriented and -driven professionals will want to have continuous involvement in shaping the interaction of professionals on the team as well as the organized system within which it works. There are proven techniques to enhance communication and collaboration, and there are great satisfactions in successful collegial work. The drive to excellence in professional service must now include a drive to work with any and all others who can enhance clinical outcomes. To the tenets of competence—the commitment and caring that have guided doctors and nurses for years—we must now add the capacity to work in integrated collegial teams. Although this chapter on service and collaboration is naturally focused upon the caregivers and health care teams, the patient-centered movement has presented us with the reality of the patient as a member of the team. As this reality becomes more commonplace, patients and health care professionals alike will have to contribute as much as they can to team morale, trust, support, and barrier-free communication.

Chapter 8

Three Paradigms for Education and Practice

Simply put, the functions of the health care professions fall into three categories: preventing, curing, and caring. Creating a more virtuous American health care system requires that health care professionals and society at large consider what should be expected in each category and in the balance of all three.

The Population-based Public Health Paradigm

Prevention, of course, implies efforts to help motivate individuals to adopt healthy lifestyles. It also refers in large part to the public health functions of populationwide initiatives such as fluoridation of the water supply, lowered speed limits, smoking cessation, mandatory immunization programs, and communicable disease surveillance practices. Prevention implies a population-based approach rooted in the science of epidemiology, which we may refer to as the population-based public health paradigm. Clearly, of all the major health professions, some will be more active than others in health promotion and disease prevention efforts. Some physicians, nurses, and dentists will join a legion of trained public health professionals in dedicating all their professional lives to public health. All physicians, nurses, and dentists, however, will need to be knowledgeable about and publicly supportive of important public health initiatives and activities.

The Reductionist Biomedical Paradigm

Curing is what most people think most physicians are doing most of the time. For the past fifty years, clinicians have been armed with a growing arsenal of technical interventions, which have emanated from the nation's extraordinary investments in basic and applied biomedical science. This arsenal has become so pervasive, so effective, and so alluring—both to patients and practitioners—that the profession may have fallen prey to the technologic imperative and lost sight of the healing impact of the physician, dentist, and nurse as therapeutic persons in their own right. The curative mode, rooted in the reductionist biomedical paradigm, rests on a disease-focused view wherein practitioners attempt to understand the molecular defect causing a disease and determine precise molecular cures. The ongoing genetic revolution stands as the latest expression of this paradigm, promising powerful new products and techniques in both the curative and preventive arenas.

But this disease-oriented paradigm has led to a dehumanization of some of what clinicians do, a minimization of the value of caring, and a scientifically unjustified dismissal of the placebo effect. It also underrates how physicians, nurses, and others can help people cope with incurable diseases, chronic suffering, and the wrenching problems that now often surround the end of life. The reductionist biomedical paradigm doesn't deal well with these matters, motivating at least some practitioners to use other avenues of approach.

The Biopsychosocial Paradigm

The biopsychosocial paradigm, espoused most clearly by psychiatrist George Engel,[1] provides an intellectual construct that addresses these matters. It identifies the disciplines that inform the techniques and strategies of human interaction necessary for the physician or any other caregiver to serve most effectively as a healer. Engel, Havens,[2] Eisenberg,[3] and Kleinman,[4] among others, have written extensively about the interface between culture, belief, the interpersonal strategies of the clinician, and the healing of the illness afflicting the whole person as well as the molecular disease afflicting his or her organ systems.

It is my personal belief that today's health profession student should understand and work with all three paradigms and make a personal synthesis of them. Alternatively, clinicians who work fundamentally within one paradigm should endeavor to achieve a balance of tolerance and respect for the other two.

Although the future rests upon a successful synthesis of and/or a creative interrelationship among the three paradigms, students may find that some of their professors seem too narrowly locked into one paradigm. Some faculty, most concerned with population-based approaches to reduce the burden of illness on society, will tend to scorn the feeble contribution of much of high-tech medicine in favor of improving overall societal health status. These people might benefit from a more sympathetic exploration of what I referred to earlier as the epidemiology of hope: the hope that so many Americans hold dear for revival or repair if disaster strikes them. The epidemiology of hope has social benefit. Many take pride in the amount of resources we commit to giving people another chance at life when other societies might abandon them. I am proud of America for that. Molecularly oriented, technology-based physicians might also seek bridges to other paradigms, perhaps by incorporating into their caregiving teams some people who possess skills from the biopsychosocial and prevention realms.

Those who do not build bridges among paradigms may be ill equipped to deliver the best care. For example, some psychiatrists and other mental health professionals may work solely within the biopsychosocial paradigm and fail to appreciate the benefits of biomedicine and public health. In doing so, they risk contributing to the isolation of the mental health enterprise from the rest of the health caregiving effort. Similarly, reductionists who fail to respect the theory behind mental health practice magnify an unnecessary gulf between "scientific" doctors and psychiatrists and psychologists.

During the last three decades, those who administer family medicine programs have led the way in creating links among the three paradigms. Swimming against the reductionist tide of the majority of medical school faculty colleagues, they have focused on a more integrative and holistic approach to care. In recent years, I have sensed that a growing cadre of faculty from across the spectrum of specialties, especially younger faculty, see medicine and health care more broadly. Furthermore, serious efforts are being made to bring public health, medicine, and the other health science professional disciplines together at both the educational and practice levels, just as some stronger initiatives are being developed to train health professionals in interprofessional collegial teams.

The following table outlines the disciplines that inform the three paradigms and the techniques and strategies that flow from each. There is too much here for any planned formal educational program to cover. Because role-modeling among medical/public health faculty tends to focus on only one of the paradigms, students need the independence of purpose and stubbornness of nature to pursue their own educations. At the same time, they must prudently negotiate the obstacle course of requirements on their way to being credentialed as a science-based healers.

	Population-based Public Health	Reductionist Biomedical	Biopsychosocial
Conceptual Basis	The health status of the population must be the subject of analysis if we are to measure and understand trends in our people's well-being.	This biomolecular paradigm rests upon the principles of modern reductionism and seeks the molecular basis for disease states and molecular cures.	There is a science to healing humans through human interaction and there are sciences that inform effective communication.
Core Academic Disciplines	Epidemiology Sociology Anthropology Political science Demography Economics Ethics	Molecular biology Chemistry Physics Mathematics Physiology Microbiology Immunology Genetics Ethics	Psychology Communication science Neuropsychiatry Sociology Anthropology Arts and liberal arts Ethics
Relative Importance to Preventing, Curing, and Caring	Crucial importance to health promotion and disease prevention strategies and research priorities. Important in measuring impact of curative interventions.	Crucial importance to understanding disease and therapy, forming the bases of many specialties. Growing importance to prevention; e.g., vaccines and mapping genetic risks.	Of most importance to curative medicine with lesser but significant relevance to prevention behavior and health promotion strategizing.
The Role of the Clinician and/or Clinical Health Care Team	To promote health and encourage behavior change, attempting to reduce risk factors like smoking and hypertension before they cause disease; to promote an environment for healthful living.	To focus on the physiologic symptoms of the patient and to match treatment with the molecular basis of the disease in the context of the patient's situation and desires.	To use the interview to collect objective information and measurements, as well as to learn more about what illness means to the individual and the capacity to cope with adversity. The integrity of these interactions builds trust, enhances compliance, and promotes patient self-healing.

There is more. There is a matter of commitment to human service, and the question of the appropriate perpetuation of a special subset of the society charged with being the chief providers of health care. In many specialties, its members receive extraordinary rewards and social standing. We ask this group, our physicians, to carry the torch of hope and the tools of therapy for those who become ill. We also ask them to initiate policies and programs that enhance and sustain the population's health status and reduce the nation's overall burden of illness and disease. Are these health professionals doing something special after all? If so, what are their social contracts? What do they profess and promise to society? This brings us to the issues of covenants and commitments in the next chapter.

But before we go there, I should let you know what has governed my own sense of work, family, and values and no doubt shaped my biases about covenantal relationships and social contracts at the professional level. At 7:30 a.m. one September day in 1958, as I drove down Sacramento Street not far from Harvard Square, I saw her standing outside the front door of her apartment, a huge bag of books in her arms and wearing dungarees and no makeup. Something told me she was the sister of a friend who was waiting for me to take her on my regular drive across the Charles River into Boston to get to the Harvard Medical School campus. Within a week, after the pheromones had worked their magic, I told Rex Jamison, an equally unmarried classmate, that I had met the person who would, if I had anything to do with it, become my future wife. I was entering the clinical years of medical school and Ruth was beginning her doctoral program in anatomy and the medical sciences. When we met we were both engaged in long and ambitious educational programs. We have spent the last half century working together. Hopefully we have added to each other's professional interests while seeking the quasi–Holy Grail of achieving individual satisfaction in related medical fields and in family life.

Our two daughters, Faith and Grace, eventually decided they had heard enough about medicine and science. Respectively, they have turned to environmental law, and organizational psychology and business. They have been anchors and rudders for us at various times, and we remain very close as a third generation has arrived.

Ruth was the second of four siblings; her father was of Russian-Lithuanian descent and her mother's roots were from Norway. Her father was a journalist early on and a businessperson later in life; her mother taught reading skills in public schools. Both completed college with a BA. Ruth's older sister got her PhD in economics under John Galbraith at Harvard, is an international expert on Russian economics and professor at the University of Washington in Seattle. Ruth got her MA in the medical sciences and finished her PhD at the University of Washington while I was being trained in internal medicine there. After the first two sisters were born, there was a twelve-year hiatus before the two younger siblings arrived. They must have absorbed some of the same familial stuff, because the brother became a physician with a PhD in genetics and the youngest sister a doctoral-prepared China expert who has spent most of her career working for the U.S. government. I must add that in all my years in higher education, I have never known of such a striking familial performance as Ruth's and her siblings'.

Sometimes our family moved because I had a new job, and a couple of times because Ruth did. Given Ruth's stature in her field and our having the same first initial, I often said that I only got tenure here or a position there because people thought they were hiring her. This was not as much of a joke as my ego occasionally would have liked. Many times people came up to me, after I had given a talk about medical education or administration, and said, "I admired your paper on the fine structure of the salt-secreting gland of the spiny dogfish, *Squalus acanthias*," or praised some other article of Ruth's. I never let on that there was a mistake and always said something like, "Thank you. I was glad to be able to do that work, but I've moved on now." When I was medical director at the University of Washington and looked about twelve years old in my senior colleagues' eyes, a committee on a new laboratory building met across the hall from my office. I was having a grand time on this committee, because I had never been involved in that sort of thing and was learning a lot. I also thought my inclusion meant that people were taking me seriously, and this was very reassuring. At the third meeting I realized that Ruth was the R. Bulger the committee wanted. When I informed the committee chair, he immediately released me from further attendance and Ruth took my, that is to say, her rightful, place.

Ruth and I have often noted that we wouldn't have traded any of it for other occupations. The opportunities to be involved in activities aimed at teaching and helping others develop have been priceless for us. We have tried to express a balance between our work and family lives, as everyone must. I believe this is very important for health professionals, if they are to fulfill their various covenants and commitments. Working together and individually was the way it was in the beginning and in the intervening years for us, and that is the way it still is!

Now let's turn to those covenants and commitments.

Chapter 9

Covenants, Commitment, and Tragic Choices

I will look upon him who shall have taught me this art even as one of my parents. I will share my substance with him, and I will supply his necessities, if he be in need. I will regard his offspring even as my own brethren and I will teach them this art, if they would learn it, without fee or covenant. I will impart this art by precept, by lecture and by every mode of teaching, not only to my own sons but to sons of him who has taught me, and to disciples bound by covenant and oath, according to the law of medicine.

The regimen I adopt shall be for the benefit of my patients according to my ability and judgment, and not for their hurt or for any wrong. I will give no deadly drug to any, though it be asked of me, nor will I counsel such, and especially I will not aid a woman to procure an abortion. Whatsoever house I enter, there will I go for the benefit of the sick, refraining from all wrongdoing or corruption, and especially from any seduction of male or female, of bond or free. Whatsoever things I see or hear concerning the life of men, in my

attendance on the sick or even apart therefrom, which ought
not to be noised abroad, I will keep silence thereon, counting
such things to be as sacred secrets.

Hippocratic Oath

Generations of medical students have taken the Hippocratic oath
upon graduation from medical school. This distillation of the teach-
ings of the father of medicine has endured for a remarkable period of
time: it was recorded some four hundred years before Christ. Although historians largely agree that the oath was not written by Hippocrates himself but by his followers after his death, the oath is
consistent with his known writings in its distinctive combination of
humanistic concern and practical wisdom—an emphasis that has inspired and guided many a physician. The Hippocratic oath remains
meaningful for me precisely because of its highly personal expression
of the basic concept of devotion to people and a desire to serve them.

The Hippocratic oath holds much wisdom even for modern
physicians and other clinicians. But many have called for reinterpret-
ing the oath in light of current knowledge and needs. Our society's
medical knowledge base and health care needs have indeed changed
over the centuries, especially in the past seventy-five years. Medicine
has become enormously complex, and as a consequence the roles that
physicians play have multiplied. Physicians these days not only carry
on general patient care, but also may become highly trained specialists; research scientists; teachers; administrators concerned with medical education, delivery of health services, or organizing our vast
biomedical research efforts; or various combinations of some or all of
the above. The Hippocratic oath seems no longer to capture all the responsibilities and obligations of physicians. According to physician
and philosopher Edmund Pellegrino, "In a simpler world, that ethic
long sufficed to guide the physician in his service to patient and
community. Today, the intersection of medicine with contemporary

science, technology, social organization, and changed human values have revealed significant missing dimensions in the ancient ethic."[1]

Among the aspects of the Hippocratic oath that society generally sees as outdated are its notions about medical training and eligibility for it. The oath asserts that doctors should teach medicine to their sons, their teachers' sons, and disciples who live "according to the law of medicine." Given the complexity of modern medicine and the structure of modern society, teaching by apprenticeship "without fee or covenant" is no longer possible, The male bias of the Hippocratic oath has long since become outmoded. Over the past fifty years, American schools have more than doubled their output of medical graduates, with the percentage of women medical graduates moving from around 5 percent to roughly 50 percent.

Thus far, efforts to increase the representation of racial minorities in medicine have been successful only to a limited extent. The numbers of black and Hispanic medical students are slowly rising in American schools, and foreign medical school graduates in our graduate residency programs have produced a steady infusion of new, ethnically diverse physicians. Because American medical school graduates can fill only about 70 percent of available first-year residency slots, the other slots are available for foreign medical graduates who can qualify. American medical schools' recent moves to increase the number of matriculating students will likely gradually reduce available residency slots for those trained abroad.

Although the Hippocratic oath will surely remain a unifying force for physicians worldwide, it cannot alone answer the need for unifying, or at least compatible, covenants among the increasingly varied health care professions. Over the past fifty years, the number of persons involved in providing health care has expanded along with new kinds of providers, such as occupational therapists, respiratory therapists, nurse practitioners, and radiologic technicians. Technological developments and changing health care needs have made it necessary to train nonphysician providers in broader areas of skills and responsibilities. As we enter the twenty-first century, more than one hundred distinct health professions contribute to the health care enterprise.

Several other circumstances, including new ethical dilemmas, have drawn modern medicine away from its Hippocratic traditions. Biomedical research involving human subjects, for example, has challenged the idea that physicians may only use their skills to benefit those in their care. When physicians become involved in placebo-controlled trials, the rigid requirements of the scientific protocol create several potential disadvantages to the people who participate as research subjects. In a similar vein, the notion of the physician as a benevolent and paternalistic figure who makes all the decisions for the patient is inconsistent with today's educated health care consumer. Informed consent was simply a nonissue in Hippocrates' time. There have also been changes in public and medical attitudes toward abortion and euthanasia that might make it difficult for today's physician to honor the portions of the oath proscribing these procedures.

Some have argued that the most important reason to update the Hippocratic oath is its lack of attention to the responsibilities of the medical profession as a whole. The tension between the interests of individuals and those of communities—so central to today's stormy health reform debate—is not acknowledged in the oath, which focuses exclusively on the responsibilities of physicians to individual patients. Dr. Pellegrino comments on the significance of this notion of communal responsibility when he writes: "Society supports the doctor in the expectation that he will direct himself to socially relevant health problems, not just those he finds interesting or remunerative. The commitment to social egalitarianism demands a greater sensitivity to social ethics than is to be found in traditional codes."[2]

Ethicist William May, in his book *The Physician's Covenant: Images of the Healer in Medical Ethics*, agrees with Pellegrino. May describes several images that capture the ways in which society perceives the physician (and in which physicians may perceive themselves). One of these images is what May calls the "covenanter." As covenanters, physicians owe a debt for their education both to society and to the patients who provide opportunities to "practice" on them. In return for public support and public trust, the physician as covenanter reciprocates with service, fidelity, accountability, and responsibility for distribution of basic services. Each of May's images of the healer provides an interesting window on the roles and responsibilities of the physician (see below); you may recognize these images embedded in the earlier chapters of this book. May has skillfully and concisely captured the healer in his choice of images, producing a most valuable book for those just entering, as well as for those already well established in, the healing professions.[3]

Pellegrino and May each argue that physicians have a covenantal relationship with society and cannot absolve themselves from responsibility for deficiencies in distribution, quality, and accessibility of care to the poor and disenfranchised. These deficiencies are widespread today. They are examples of the complexities of modern society that the Hippocratic oath, even with its ethical sensibilities and high moral tone, does not adequately address.

William F. May's Images of the Healer

Fighter—The healer is a fighter against death. Patients prize a kind of military intelligence, tactical brilliance, self-confidence, and stamina in the healer. The language of war dominates the understanding of disease (e.g., cancer "invades," hearts are "attacked") and shapes the healer's response (e.g., searching for a magic "bullet," utilizing an "armamentarium" of drugs).

Parent—The healer's role is to nurture and reassure patients and shelter them from the powers that are hurting them. Kindness rather than candor is the chief moral virtue expected of the healer. As between parent and child, the healer's relationship is characterized by compassion (e.g., shared suffering) and self-expenditure (i.e., the imbalance of knowledge and power define the healer as the giver and the patient as the receiver).

Technician—Excellent technical performance becomes the effective center of the professional ethic; the healer finds satisfaction in service, but technology and technical performance supply his or her ultimate justification. The healer's white lab coat points to the scientific origin of medical authority and hints at the body mechanic at work. The criteria for admission to medical school and the grading system that prevails there emphasize the preeminent place of technical performance in the formation and career of the professional.

Covenanter—Healers have distinctive obligations to their patients and to their teachers (as in the Hippocratic oath). Patients effectively "teach" healers by allowing healers to "practice" on them. Healers also owe a debt to the society that supports their training; they owe competence, accountability, the courage to hold fellow professionals accountable, and responsibility for the distribution of basic services. Service and fidelity are chief moral virtues of the healer. The patient is a bonded partner in pursuit of health.

Teacher—The healer respects patients' intelligence and power of self-determination. To be an effective teacher requires a kind of imagination that permits the healer to enter into the life circumstances of the patient-learner to reckon with the difficulties the patient faces in acquiring, assimilating, and acting on what he or she needs to know. Those skills are particularly important in preventive, rehabilitative, chronic, and terminal care. They often go unrewarded in third-party payment systems and receive little attention in medical schools and residency programs.

The Hippocratic Oath's Enduring Appeal and Modern Alternatives

Despite its jagged-edge fit in the world of modern medicine, the Hippocratic oath endures. There have been several attempts to create new oaths, but the majority of graduating medical students still prefer to take the Hippocratic oath, even though several of its propositions have little or no modern relevance. Perhaps this is due in part to the appeal of a spiritual link with the world of ancient Greece, a feeling that speaking the words of Hippocrates and his early disciples connects one in a special way to the four-thousand-year-old roots of Western scientific medicine—and to the historical prestige of a select professional group. The oath allows one to touch a tradition that transcends personal interests and rivets attention on meaningful superordinate goals.

Certainly, the Hippocratic oath has also persisted because of the premises at its core: competence and caring. As I have tried to argue, these foundational Hippocratic values are still at the heart of modern physicianhood, even if they don't cover all the necessary bases in twenty-first century America.

In 1988, I made my own attempt to fashion a version of the Hippocratic oath that reflects the enduring appeal of the original, but that also addresses the complexities of modern life and can guide activities that otherwise may become hopelessly complex, bureaucratic, and impersonal, as follows:

The Oath of the Modern Hippocrates

- By all that I hold highest, I promise my patients competence, integrity, candor, personal commitment to their best interests, compassion, and absolute discretion and confidentiality within the law.
- I shall do by my patients as I would be done by; shall obtain consultation whenever I or they desire, shall include them to the extent they wish in all important decisions, and shall minimize suffering whenever a cure cannot be obtained, understanding that a dignified death is an important goal in everyone's life.

- I shall try to establish a friendly relationship with my patients and shall accept each one in a nonjudgmental manner, appreciating the validity and worth of different value systems and according to each person a full measure of human dignity.

- I shall charge only for my professional services and shall not profit financially in any other way as a result of the advice and care I render my patients.

- I shall provide advice and encouragement for my patients in their efforts to sustain their own health.

- I shall work with my profession to improve the quality of medical care and to improve the public's health, but I shall not let any lesser public or professional consideration interfere with my primary commitment to provide the best and most appropriate care available to each of my patients.

- To the extent I live by these precepts, I shall be a worthy physician.[4]

The same year, Pellegrino and Thomasma argued for the concept of beneficence as the central value in patient care. With their analysis, they presented an excellent modern oath, even as they pointed out that oaths are not sufficient:

A Physician's Commitment to Promoting the Patient's Good

I promise to fulfill the obligations I voluntarily assume by my profession to heal, and to help those who are ill. My obligations rest in the special vulnerability of the sick and the trust they must ultimately place in me and my professional competence. I therefore bind myself to the good of my patient in its many dimensions as the first principle of my professional ethics. In recognition of this bond, I accept the following obligations from which only the patient or the patient's valid surrogates can release me:

1. To place the good of the patient at the center of my professional practice and, when the gravity of the situation demands, above my own self-interest.

2. To possess and maintain the competence in knowledge and skill I profess to have.

3. To recognize the limitations of my competence and to call upon my colleagues in all the health professions whenever my patient's needs require.

4. To respect the values and beliefs of my colleagues in the other health professions and to recognize their moral accountability as individuals.

5. To care for all who need my help with equal concern and dedication, independent of their ability to pay.

6. To act primarily in behalf of my patient's best interests, and not primarily to advance social, political, or fiscal policy, or my own interests.

7. To respect my patient's moral right to participate in the decisions that affect him or her, by explaining clearly, fairly, and in language understood by the patient the nature of his or her illness, together with the benefits and dangers of the treatments I propose to use.

8. To assist my patients to make choices that coincide with their own values or beliefs, without coercion, deception or duplicity.

9. To hold in confidence what I hear, learn, and see as a necessary part of my care of the patient, except when there is a clear, serious, and immediate danger of harm to others.

10. Always to help, even if I cannot cure, and when death is inevitable, to assist my patient to die according to his or her own life plans.

11. Never to participate in direct, active, conscious killing of a patient, even for reasons of mercy, or at the request of the state, or for any other reason.

12. To fulfill my obligation to society to participate in public policy decisions affecting the nation's health by providing leadership, as well as expert and objective testimony.

13. To practice what I preach, teach, and believe and, thus, to embody the foregoing principle in my professional life.[5]

Seven colleagues from across the country—Ralph Crawshaw, Edmund Pellegrino, Christine Cassel, David Rogers, George Lundberg, Lonnie Bristow, and Jeremiah Barondess—and I took a different approach in 1995. After getting together intermittently, we developed the following statement, which was published that year in the May 17 issue of the *Journal of the American Medical Association*. As far as I know, it quickly dropped off anyone's radar screen.

Patient-Physician Covenant

Medicine is, at its center, a moral enterprise grounded in a covenant of trust. This covenant obliges physicians to be competent and to use their competence in the patient's best interests. Physicians, therefore, are both intellectually and morally obliged to act as advocates for the sick wherever their welfare is threatened and for their health at all times.

Today, this covenant of trust is significantly threatened. From within, there is growing legitimization of the physician's materialistic self-interest; from without for-profit forces press the doctor into the role of commercial agent to enhance the profitability of health care organizations. Such distortions of the doctor's responsibility degrade the doctor/patient relationship that is the central element and structure of medical care. To capitulate to these alterations of the trust relationship is to significantly alter the doctor's role as healer, carer, helper and advocate for the sick and for the health of all.

By its traditions and very nature, medicine is a special kind of human activity—one which cannot be pursued effectively without the virtues of humility, honesty, intellectual integrity, compassion and effacement of excessive self-interest. These traits mark doctors as members of a moral community dedicated to something other than its own self-interest.

Our first obligation must be to serve the good of those persons who seek our help and trust us to provide it. Physicians, as physicians, are not, and must never be, commercial entrepreneurs, gate-closers, or agents of fiscal policy that runs counter to our trust. Any defection from the primacy of the patient's well-being places the patient at risk by treatment which may compromise quality of or access to medical care.

We believe the medical profession must reaffirm the primacy of its obligation to the patient through national, state, and local professional societies, our academic, research, and hospital organizations, and especially through personal behavior. As advocates for the promotion of health and support of the sick, we are called upon to discuss, defend and promulgate effective medical care by every means available. Only by caring and advocating for the patient can the integrity of our profession be affirmed.

Thus we honor our covenant of trust with patients.

Since these covenantal statements were written, times have continued to change. There has been growing recognition of the value and often the necessity of health care professionals delivering care in teams. Personal commitment of the physician to her or his patient may have been sufficient when the medical team averaged one doctor and three other professionals. This is no longer the case, now that the health care team draws from over a hundred distinct health professions. Not counted in this total are the variety of others who have a role in health care decision making, including health system administrators, third-party payers, and patients and their families. Collaboration among the various players has taken on an importance that Hippocrates never could have imagined.

No modern covenant for health care providers would thus be complete without acknowledging the need for collaboration among the members of the health care team. In the complicated and sometimes perplexing arena of high-tech health care, only groups of providers, functioning as a competent and caring team, can deliver high-quality, highly effective care. As an intended supplement to the oaths of their individual professions, colleagues from dentistry, nursing, pharmacy, and medicine accordingly developed the following covenant:

Health Professions Covenant

As a health care professional dedicated to enhancing the well-being of individuals and communities, I am committed to achieving and sustaining the highest level of professional competence, to fulfilling my responsibilities with compassion for patients' suffering, and to helping patients make their own informed choices about health care whenever possible. Recognizing that effective health promotion, disease prevention, and curative and long-term care are products of the combined efforts of teams of health professionals, I pledge collaboration with all of my colleagues similarly committed to meeting the health care needs of individuals and their communities. Further, I will work within my profession to encourage placement of the patient's and the public's interests above the self-interests of my individual profession.

The Association of Academic Health Centers recommended this brief amendment to health professionals' different oaths in the first few years of the twenty-first century. Not long after that, the CEOs of most major health professions' educational associations also recommended it, and several academic health centers have used it at their graduation ceremonies. Interestingly, the only demurral came from the medical school deans, whose council sent the message that there was nothing in the Health Professions Covenant that wasn't already well covered in the Hippocratic oath. Go figure! It is my hope that health professionals at least consider incorporating a statement like this one into the covenantal ceremonies in which they participate before entering the world of practice. Fulfillment of the traditional tenets of health care espoused in the major oaths taken by graduates into the individual professions, including the ancient Hippocratic oath, increasingly depends upon teamwork and collaboration.

Institutional Values

Modern life generally involves working, studying, or pursuing other activities within public and private institutions. As suggested in previous chapters, our society is beginning to appreciate how an institution's values can have far-reaching effects on those within and outside its walls. For example, a health care institution undermines its credibility if it does not take tangible steps to improve the health of its own employees through such measures as smoking cessation, diet, and exercise programs.

Health care institutions that place disproportionate value on the number of patient visits their providers accumulate, the number of dollars saved or dollars earned, and other economic measures and goals run the risk of compromising care by placing too many constraints on clinicians and clinical teams. When rationing of technology and caregivers' time characterizes an institution's ethos, commitment to service and collaboration in meeting the needs of patients all too often can get lost in the shuffle. Without time and without some flexibility in time management, it almost doesn't matter how committed providers are to service and collaboration; there is no place for these endeavors.

A revealing perspective on the interaction of individual, institutional, and professional values emerges from a 1973 landmark study of senior divinity students at Princeton Theological Seminary. The researchers, John Darley and C. Daniel Batson, contrived an elaborate experiment to study people's willingness to help someone in need. The experiment might not be repeatable today because it involved deceiving its subjects.

Near the end of the semester, the divinity students were to meet individually with an instructor to record a prepared talk. One group had been assigned to write a talk about the parable of the Good Samaritan; the others were asked to make presentations about careers in the ministry. On the day of the experiment, the students were directed one by one to a nearby building where the talks would be taped. The students were given one of three time constraints: "Hurry, you're already late!," "They're ready for you now—please go right over," or "It will be a few minutes before they are ready for you, but you'd best head over."

On the way, each student encountered a young man writhing on the lawn in pain. The man was actually a paid trained observer playing the role of the modern counterpart of the man encountered millennia ago by the Good Samaritan. Besides acting, his job was to record which students stopped, what they did when they stopped, and how long they stayed.

Of the group as a whole, 40 percent offered some form of aid to the man in pain, with no difference between those about to give a talk on the Good Samaritan and those about to talk on careers in the clergy. The only variable that correlated with whether or not students stopped to offer assistance was the time expectation they thought they were facing. Broken down according to time constraints, 63 percent of the "unhurried" group, 45 percent of the "somewhat hurried" group, and only 10 percent of the "hurried" group stopped to aid the apparent sufferer. There was no escaping the conclusion, wrote the authors, that the divinity students decided whether or not to care for a stranger in distress based on their perceived time pressure.[6] The study did not determine to what degree the personal priority of completing their studies successfully motivated the students' decisions, but it clearly indicates how even subtle institutional priorities, in the form of the different messages about time, influenced their readiness to fulfill the obvious imperative for a minister of tending to someone in need.

Kenneth Ludmerer's two books on the history of American medical education, *Learning to Heal*[7] and *Time to Heal*,[8] show how the tragic choice between time and caring occurs every day in our hospitals, clinics, and doctors' offices. What we know about the placebo effect, taking care of those who are suffering, and the healing power of words indicates that rationing of caregivers' time can have serious negative consequences for patients. As we work to reform the health care system with potential cost-effective improvements, we should recognize that taking away the tools of communication, companionship, compassion, and shared decision making will do more harm than good. Instead, we must enhance the tools of the healing relationship between clinicians and patients and between institutions and patients.

Together with the growth in numbers and kinds of health professionals, the ways in which our health care system already rations caregivers' time (based on financial constraints) and patients' access to health care (based on their ability to pay) point to two complex issues. How, and how much, should we pay doctors, nurses, and the legion of other professionals who have joined the health care team?

How do we predict how many of each of the various professionals we need, if indeed it is possible to make such predictions rationally?

In these economic hard times, many people question what they feel are excessive charges by physicians and hospitals, pointing to the fee-for-service mechanism as the problem. Fee-for-service and universal health care are not incompatible, however. Physicians in Canada and some Western European countries are paid on a fee-for-service basis. Anyone who has a Medicare card and incurs medical bills sees the following on the regular reports: what the doctor or hospital billed for the service rendered, followed sequentially by the dollar amount Medicare approved (often less than what was billed by significant amounts); the dollar amount Medicare actually paid (often a still smaller figure); and a final figure showing the dollars the physician or hospital may yet bill the patient. Thus, one can see that Medicare has some tools available to control health care payments and to carry out the negotiations in public.

The first figure on the medical bill represents what would be asked if Medicare were not involved, and the final figure what the doctor or hospital hopes to receive directly from the patient or from Medicare-supplementing private insurance. In practice, doctors and hospitals do not count on patients' paying the non-Medicare amount out of pocket, but private insurers do a brisk business selling Medicare-supplementing insurance packages to employers and individuals. The insured person gets more of the initial bill paid and a larger number to provide as a co-pay, and the insurance company gets its 20 percent charge to manage the account.

Our problem is not so much fee-for-service as it is our particular financing scheme and the absence of controls on overutilization of services. When people are upset about physicians' fees and incomes, it is important to realize that the incomes of general physicians, family physicians, and pediatricians are by most people's standards not excessive and frequently could be considered too low by some.

Advanced practice nurses are also now operating in the private practice, fee-for-service mode as are some physician associates, and their incomes are reaching the same range as general physicians. If the quality is equal, that is as it should be. Finally, it should be noted that salaried positions are becoming more popular among physicians, because they feel freer to practice medicine and less bound up in business management.

I believe that some form of public option, along with government subsidies for those who cannot afford to buy insurance, will force the insurance companies into offering less expensive and competitive coverage for the care we all need. This in turn will reduce dollars available for excessively expensive operations and unnecessary tests. The biggest difficulty arises from physician ownership of hospitals and related patient-care facilities and businesses, ranging from CAT scanners to lithotripters to laboratory facilities. Self-referral and conflicts of interest in such situations endanger patients' trust in individual physicians and the entire profession and health care team.

Regarding health workforce size planning and prognostication, I have lived through several cyclical periods where the supposed experts, including me, joined together to declare that the country had too many or too few dentists, doctors, or nurses. In almost every case, except in shortages of dentists and nurses, we had it wrong. The most striking example was when the medical schools were holding fast to their existing class sizes in anticipation of improved efficiency via managed care. Osteopathic schools, sensing the unmet demand of potential students for more places to enter the medical professions, expanded quite dramatically. They turned out to be right and we were wrong, because too many variables affect need in the marketplace five years out to do anything but let students know the realities of the moment in terms of available positions.

One thing our country and other developed countries need to change is addressing shortages of physicians and nurses by taking them from third world countries. This has disastrous effects on the health of the third world. The BBC reported in October 2009 that of two hundred doctors recently trained in Malawi, only fifty remained in the country. Referring to the fact that Malawian women die in childbirth at a rate fourteen times that of women in developed countries, Dorothy Ngoma, head of the main nursing union in Malawi, told the BBC, "We have more Malawian doctors in Manchester, [England,] than in the whole of Malawi. There are more than two hundred of them. Imagine if those doctors came back and spread out across our hospitals here, how many women's lives would be saved?"[9]

Such situations, common throughout the third world, suggest that developed countries should expand medical education at home, creating more opportunities for their own people to become physicians and nurses, and support both medical education and medical careers in developing countries.

Suffice it to say that pay scales for physicians in comparison to other health professionals will remain a complicated and controversial issue in America. So will the much debated impact of immigration on population growth and labor supply and demand in the health care sector and the rest of the economy. America has been struggling to come to terms with these issues, and I predict it will continue to do so for some time.

It is important for the next generation of physicians, dentists, psychologists, nurses, pharmacists, and other caregivers to continually reexamine the validity, as well as the cultural and personal meanings, of their professional oaths and covenants to themselves and their patients. The alternative is contractual health care restricting what will be done in exchange for what—this much and no more! Despite the challenges our health care enterprise faces in meeting the vast and varied health needs of today's society, health care offers among the most rewarding careers available. If this book has conveyed anything substantive to the younger reader, I hope the message includes the extraordinary breadth of interest and scholarship open to health professionals, which continually challenges them to keep learning from a wide array of disciplines and experiences. Clinical health care offers the opportunity to marry the worlds of action, emotion, mind, and spirit. Little more can be asked of a profession, and the country and the world will always need dedicated health workers!

Chapter 10

Measuring American Health Care with Human Values

Without research, there is no hope!
Paul G. Rogers[1]

Thinking about the future is only useful and interesting
if it affects what we do today.
James Robertson, futurist

We have the best sick care system in the world.
The problem is that we don't have good health care.
Dr. Joycelyn Elders,
former U.S. Surgeon General

I was accused in the 1930s of being a Communist for
carrying a placard declaring that all health care should
be free! It was all a horrible lie! What the placard actually said was ALL EFFECTIVE HEALTH CARE SHOULD BE
FREE! That left 95% of health care for the capitalistic
systems.
Archie Cochrane, PhD[2]

No matter what we wish or predict for the future, none of us knows what will happen. The best we can do is learn from history and what is going on now to help us formulate the next steps for our nation and our world.

Our future is happening to us right now, if we can recognize it. The most effective approaches to influencing the course of our health care future will surely arise from understanding our history, our cultural values, and the realities of the current environment. We should begin by examining trends, identifying transformational forces, and adhering to our core American values. Then we should identify the elements of our existing health care system in terms of those factors. Finally, we should develop measures and evaluative tools to determine the effectiveness of the twenty-first-century health care sector as it functions in our society.

I propose that our society should ultimately require our health care sector to provide mercy, justice, hope, and individual autonomy for all our citizens. In health care, mercy and justice may be expressed better by referring to compassion and equity. Most observers would surely agree that individual autonomy, equity, compassion, and hope are core American values. Whatever our society is doing and shall do in the future, we must measure our health care against these four basic values.

Living up to these values can lead the way to establishing a typically American version of health care for all, an optimal and improving health status for all, and a tangible demonstration of the civilizing effects of our great 230-year-old national experiment with democracy.

Where Are We Now?

We remain in a state of considerable confusion, with enormous pressure building to fix our health care system. Most of us recognize it is too costly, poorly organized, and inequitably distributed. But it is of tremendous value in saving lives, extending quality of life for many, and leading the world in applying modern science to health promotion, disease prevention, diagnosis, and treatment. Trying to grade the health care industry in terms of the four basic American values, I would give us a B- in autonomy, a B+ in hope, a C+ in mercy, and a D in justice. Having said this, I have to admit that such an assessment is of no lasting value. Without data organized to measure health care performance against our fundamental social values, it is and must remain a personal opinion.

With that thought, and James Robertson's words at the head of this chapter in mind, I end this book with a sample evaluative model designed to produce consistent and repeatable measurements of health care in terms of our basic values and the cost, quality, and effectiveness of specific treatments. Before we get to that, however, we might return to my grades and use them to summarize where we are now in U.S. health care and where we want to go. Our overall goal should be to get an A for each of the four cardinal American health care values.

My B- grade for individual autonomy reflects my belief that the patriarchal "doctor knows best and patients must follow orders" model no longer meets the needs of most Americans. A growing legion of patients and their families bent on taking charge of their own health care decision making. Consequently, increasing numbers of physicians and other health professionals are replacing this model with one in which health professionals are consultants, advisors, and counselors to their patients, rather than their commanding officers. My B- is an honor grade, but it leaves enormous room for improvement. To improve, we need to enhance the quality of information available to patients. We also need to increase the number of people empowered through their insurance coverage to take charge of their own health and make decisions before medical emergencies occur.

I have given us a B+ for hope, because of our long history of public and private support for biomedical research. This research has produced treatments capable of bringing patients back from the brink of death. Such services are often at their best in inner-city hospitals serving whoever is injured and brought to their busy emergency rooms and trauma centers. The American people share the widespread hope that our health care system will give every injured or seriously ill person a chance to recover. But research into the serious health disparities among various segments of our population has been slow in gaining adequate support. Above all, this research indicates that early, appropriate diagnosis can save many lives in disadvantaged populations.

In this connection, President George W. Bush's administration deserves credit for continuing and increasing funding for our community health center system. This has helped address some of our inherent failings in giving hope equally to all Americans. The health research infrastructure provisions in President Barack Obama's stimulus bill promise not only a continued flow of new medicines and techniques, to address both acute and chronic illnesses, but also an improvement in our health-promoting and disease-prevention efforts. If we ensure that all citizens have health care coverage, we will have gone a long way to raising our grade on hope to an A+. An important step to this goal occurred during the first month of the Obama administration with the passage and signing of the State Children's Health Insurance Program (SCHIP) legislation, providing health care coverage to millions of previously uncovered children.

I have given us a C+ in mercy. Because most doctors now practice in groups rather than as individuals, and health care has become the product of increasingly large and complex teams of varied health professionals, the dispensation of mercy extends far beyond the reach of a lead physician or nurse. Over the past two to three decades, both acute medical and hospital care and specialist chronic care have shown significant improvements in their patient-centeredness and sensitivity to suffering. In particular we have made remarkable progress in our societal relationship to death and the ability of our systems, hospitals, and clinics to ameliorate the suffering of patients and family members coming to terms with impending death. Yet there remains a lot to do in this area, in addition to extending the reach of modern Western medicine and health care to the almost 50 million Americans without health insurance coverage and the many millions who are underinsured.

Finally, we get a D for justice and health equity. We can only improve the grade by providing universal health care. This is not simply a financing issue. It requires deciding what works and what doesn't, what should be paid for and what shouldn't, and how to provide the human and technological resources to reach every citizen.

When Archie Cochrane made the remarks quoted at the head of this chapter, he felt there hadn't been all that much progress since he gave British health care an overall effectiveness rating of 5 percent in the late 1930s. His advocacy for what we now call evidence-based medicine has had enormous influence. The Cochrane Collaboration, his enduring worldwide legacy, is a network designed to identify effective diagnostic methods and treatments to which everyone should have access. Today, experts will differ as to whether 30 or 50 percent of what we do in health care is effective. However, there seems no doubt that in the future we shall have to require, in terms of basic health insurance for every American, that only those interventions shown to be effective be covered. This means that unproven approaches will require ongoing clinical trials of safety and effectiveness. In the meantime, they can be purchased by those who wish to spend their own money that way.

Postmodern Health Care
and the Medical Home

For me, postmodernism does not mean rejecting the Enlightenment, the scientific revolutions of the past two hundred years, or the use of logic, reason, and observation in problem solving. As I have mentioned, following Jaroslav Pelikan's lead of a couple of decades ago means rejecting the idea that pure reason offers the only way of knowing and determining our actions. Science may one day be able to reduce the wisdom and insights of great poets and prophets, and the intuitive leaps of great scientists, to logical theory and demonstration. For now community and individual life demands a broader social, cultural, and ethical dimension that embraces technical mastery and moderates its sometimes negative effects.[3]

Put another way, if we are in the business of helping people get and stay healthy, we must orient ourselves to both sides of their brains, just as we must do when we accept the challenge of helping them cope when death approaches. Postmodern health care also means broadening our horizons and scope of involvement to deal effectively with the challenges of an aging population and the growing incidence of chronic diseases.

Globalism has affected our health as well as our economies. AIDS has brought home to everyone the threat of worldwide pandemics. We have witnessed a great number of wounded and lives lost in our wars. These occurrences, as well as the advancing longevity of our populace, have dented our collective consciousness. We cannot escape the reality of suffering from chronic disease and the fact that death awaits us all. I believe these things represent a transformational force that has already had, and will continue to have, a significant effect on our health care culture.

The dramatic trend to patient-centered care reflects these developments and constitutes a transformational force on its own account.

Patient-centered care has spawned the concept of the medical home, an entity that coordinates patients' care, keeps their medical records, and enables them to act virtually as the chair of the board of their own personal health care companies. The technology already exists to make this possible.

Why shouldn't I, right now, be able to link my primary care clinician, my oncologist and cardiologist, my dentist, my eye doctor, the pharmacist, the physical therapist, and the visiting nurse, all as necessary and appropriate, to my health and medical records? Why shouldn't I be able to give access to my medical record to another specialist for a second opinion on important treatment options? Why shouldn't I be able to reach through the Internet to assess the different protocols for treatment of a particular chronic disease, like cancer or heart disease, from which I may be suffering? And why shouldn't I quickly be able to measure the economic consequences of doing A vs. B and their respective interplay with my health insurance and the impact on my out-of-pocket responsibilities? Indeed, why shouldn't I be able to tap into a data bank containing anonymized aggregations of data describing patients like me and various effective protocols for dealing with whatever might be confronting me and my doctor at the moment? Why shouldn't I be able to contact my team with a personally vexing problem and quickly resolve how to deal with it?

All these possibilities are in place or under development somewhere around us, in bits and pieces, some larger and more coordinated than others. The advance of information technology (IT) and the complexity of our increasing specialization of knowledge can take us to a new level of patient autonomy over this next decade, along with better care, less unnecessary treatment, and sustainable economics. If we don't get there, the most likely cause will be, as Walt Kelly's comics character Pogo said, "We have met the enemy and he is us." Our own fears about misuse of our personal data may trump our very deep American instinct to find the most efficient way forward.[4]

When I dealt with my own most recent serious illness, I became less concerned about the possibility of an occasional lessening of privacy. The privacy issue is the all too often unrecognized elephant in the room in relation to the vast potential of computerization in health care. We can't solve the problem here and now, it seems, and will likely have to wait until advancing technology makes us decide.

In addition to patient privacy, the obstacles to implementing the medical home plan throughout the health care system include things like the needs of multilingual patient populations. But the problems are not insurmountable. One day in the mid-1950s, the prime minister of the United Kingdom declared that exactly one year from that date, every citizen had to have signed up with a primary care physician in order to be covered by the National Health Service. One year later it was, in fact, done. Why can't we envision that one day within the next few years, an analogous announcement be made for everyone to choose a home for their electronic health and medical records, along with a primary care physician or facility of their choice? Depending on circumstances, the medical home and information-treatment hub might be a community health center, an organization like the Kaiser Permanente Health Plan, or an institution like the Mayo Clinic.

Demographics will make this a more and more compelling prospect. I believe that the flood of elderly will overwhelm the available physician workforce, and that the ranks of nurse practitioners and physician's associates will expand to fill the gap. Physicians, nurses, and other nonphysician clinicians, using telemedicine systems, will likely coordinate their services as teams to provide cost-effective preventive and medical services to the geriatric and chronic disease populations. As I write, large pharmaceutical chains are establishing "minute clinics" with physicians and other clinicians on duty seven days a week. It is not hard to believe that sometime soon, a centralized but personalized medical record will connect customers with all their various caregivers, at least as regards the drugs they take. Other dimensions of this future have already arrived in the form of patients with specific diseases forming chat groups or blogs to share problems, challenges, and best practices, often with expert physicians entering the discussions.

Those who oppose providing health insurance for every American often contrast cumbersome big government with allegedly non-bureaucratic private care. This ignores the fact, well known to most people who have private health insurance, that much private care has become at least as bureaucratic as Medicare. The debate over universal health coverage is also bedeviled by concerns about cost. For years, economists and political scientists have guesstimated that 25 to 50 percent of our health care expenditures are unnecessary. When it comes to delivering high-quality care at lower cost, both the public and private sectors offer encouraging evidence.

We also know that we can save money on treatment procedures while obtaining better patient outcomes. Longitudinal analyses of the outcomes of competing treatments can reveal which practices are most effective and, among those, which are most cost-effective. When group practices share these sorts of data, they all rapidly convert to adopting and applying the most cost-effective treatments. A decade-long effort by the American Medical Groups Association (AMGA) has shown that treatment outcome data collection and sharing can produce the highest standard of effective care in the nation for a reduction in cost of 30 percent below the national average.

With member organizations averaging around 275 physicians each, AMGA member organizations are in forty-two states and serve a total patient population of 50 million persons. Through Anceta, a separate health informatics corporation established to serve as the data bank for its members, AMGA has succeeded in protecting institutional and patient privacy while improving quality and lowering costs. The farsightedness of AMGA and its leader, Don Fisher, includes a visionary attempt, still some years from fruition, to make such data accessible to individual patients and/or practitioners, as they seek to find the best available treatments.

By far the most impressive ongoing effort to develop principles for achieving cost-effective, high-quality universal health care has been that of the National Coalition for Health Care (NCHC), founded and led for the past two decades by Dr. Henry Simmons. The NCHC's more than one hundred member organizations, including major corporations, not-for-profit health and social agencies, unions, hospitals, associations, religious groups, and others have a combined constituency of an estimated 170 million persons.

Thanks to the collective efforts and input of its member organizations, bipartisan political support, and the involvement of leading health economists and medical and public health professionals, the NCHC has developed a robust conceptual framework for universal health care coverage. The framework's basic elements, consistent with a more recent plan developed by former senators Bob Dole and Tom Daschle, include a new national entity analogous to the Federal Reserve Board. It would be empowered to determine which services and interventions are effective and cost efficient enough to be included in the health care services to be covered by mandated insurances. Operating with an inflation-adjusted national spending limit, such an entity could bring within our reach the societal moral imperative of health care for all at a reasonable cost.

Rationing, the Medical-Industrial Complex, and We the Patients

Years ago, a number of American colleagues and I visited a leading Israeli health care executive, who summarized the differences between the American and Israeli approaches to health care by saying, "You pay not to wait! We wait not to pay!" In the decades after that remark, we in America learned how to ration professional time in order not to pay so much. We are still struggling with how to sustain humanity in a time-constrained medical environment. But if it is true that you get what you pay for, it is also true that we as a society have until recently not looked carefully at the hidden costs of the system our vast health care payments have created.

When Dwight D. Eisenhower left the White House at the end of his second presidential term, he issued a dramatic warning about the self-interested agenda of what he indelibly labeled the military-industrial complex. A decade or so later, Dr. Arnold S. Relman, then the editor of the *New England Journal of Medicine*, similarly warned about the danger to society posed by the medical-industrial complex.[5] The health care industry, the largest in the country, dwarfs even the defense industry. As a nation we spend over 15 percent of gross domestic product on health care and just over 4 percent on defense. In the past few years, an array of well-documented books and articles have chronicled the corporatization of our health care.[6] There is no doubt that health care has become a big business or perhaps is better described as a huge conglomerate of big businesses, with all the attendant advantages and disadvantages.

One serious disadvantage is the economic risk facing the insured and underinsured, as well as the 47 to 50 million uninsured, from phenomenal cost escalation. In his recent bestselling book, *High Wire: The Precarious Financial Lives of American Families*, *Los Angeles Times* reporter Peter Gosselin has amply documented how even apparently adequately insured members of the middle class risk bankruptcy from health care costs, one of several de facto forms of health care rationing in our society.[7] As the health care legislation requested by President Obama slowly took shape in 2009, debate revolved more around philosophic preferences for private enterprise versus big government than around figuring out how to bring every American the security of good, affordable health care. This ensured that, whatever the immediate political outcome of health care reform might be, our health care delivery institutions, organizations, and groups of caregivers will continue to face multiple dilemmas in trying to deliver the efficient, effective, humane health care Americans want and deserve.

I believe that to an important degree, despite our oaths, covenants, and ideals, we health professionals tend to become what we measure. Therefore, at the end of this book I present an approach to measuring what we do in health care—the Organizational Therapeutic Index (OTI)—in order to reflect both what we are and what we hope to become. The OTI aims to be a balanced scorecard, a notion that has recently become very popular in management practice and theory. But my model is actually the structured report cards for students in the 1940s New York City public school system.

The front of the report card showed the student's and teacher's names. When the card was opened, the left-hand side listed four or five student behavioral characteristics, each of which had a space for the teacher to check a box for "excellent," "satisfactory," or "unsatisfactory." The righthand side listed all the subjects with spaces available for the traditional letter grades. The two most important behavioral characteristics for me were "respects the rights of others" and "works well with others." If I passed the bar on those two, whatever happened on the right side of the card didn't matter so much to my parents. When I reflect on the fact that for many years every New York City public school student through the eighth grade saw that half the report card was on behavioral and social qualities and the other on learning competence and performance, it underlines for me the importance of effective and broad value-based measures.

In the years ahead, our challenge will be to learn how to assess the human dimensions and psychological impacts of our health care enterprises, large and small, as well as the cost effectiveness and efficiency of varied treatment protocols. It is a daunting task to develop a measuring tool kit that can meet that challenge in our data-driven universe. But I believe it can be done.

Understanding the human dimensions and psychological aspects of health care will be all the more important as we necessarily leave behind an era of implicit, often inhumane health care rationing in America and enter an era of explicit, and for that reason hopefully wiser and more humane, health care rationing.

The Health Care Workforce

In addition to our shift from modernism to postmodernism, patient-centered care, and the medical home another major transforming force is the need for health professionals to respect each other's evolving roles in developing a multiplicity of subsystems of care for the future. Reaching every American will require innovative models for workforce collaboration and teamwork. For example, meeting the needs of populations (rural and urban; geriatric; or any age) trying to cope with chronic disease and disability—particularly heavy-burden disease entities like heart disease, cancer, mental illness, and behavioral compulsions, including substance dependence—as well as culturally diverse subpopulations will call for both inter- and intraprofessional team practice.

Demographers and geographers tell us there is a potential tsunamilike wave of elderly coming our way. They also say that within twenty years the extent of American cultural and racial diversity will turn every ethnic group into a minority. We can also reasonably expect that worldwide pandemics—we know not what, when, or how—will come upon or start with us. Finally, technology may set us free and help us cope, but it can be transformational in unexpectedly detrimental ways. Just mentioning the word "nanotechnology" should make the point.

The Mature Healer and the Therapeutic Institution

Public accountability looms large at American institutions today, forcing a reevaluation within many organizations of how, and how well, they are accomplishing their goals. In a number of cases, the analysis uncovers adjustments that must be made if the corporation or institution is to retain or rebuild the public's trust. The health care system is no exception. In the wake of great advances in medical science and technology, patient and clinician have developed an increased appetite for getting and giving, respectively, the most modern health care available. However, the tremendous developments in modern science that will ultimately contribute to improved health care are being constrained by the health care environment. Here issues of quality and cost vie for primacy, systems of care become ever more complex, and the sometimes disparate interests of government agencies, private insurers, and corporate health care institutions collide.

Max Weber, the influential societal theorist, taught that one purpose of society is to arrange for the distribution of available goods and that bureaucracies are needed to make such arrangements. The more widespread the task, the more centralized the means of distribution become. In the health care field, bureaucracy has increasingly separated the patient and provider, eroding the trust on which much of the clinician's status, respect, and therapeutic capacity depend. Studies tell us that patients and the public alike have lost their previous high level of faith in hospitals and physicians. The majority of Americans in health care plans suspect that the plans reward the providers for providing less costly care, frequently at the expense of quality care. Furthermore, and perhaps as a by-product, the morale of doctors and nurses has almost dropped off the radar screen.

One response to this problem that is receiving attention in health care circles is to amplify traditional covenants and agreements so they incorporate the concept of healing care. This effort focuses on the formation of the complete clinician, or what I would prefer to call the mature healer: someone in touch with the totality of a patient's needs, both physical and emotional.

As discussed in earlier chapters, many factors go into the making of the mature healer, including the embodiment of numerous medical and scientific techniques passed down through the ages. I have already mentioned, William May's five images of the complete clinician-healer: a fighter who makes war on disease; a parental figure who demonstrates compassion and benevolence; a technician who believes that technical performance is of ultimate importance; a covenanter who values responsibility, service, and fidelity; and a teacher who assists patients in developing healthy habits and coping with incurability.[8] A clinician who operates in only one of these areas is by definition incomplete.

Against a background of scientific and technical competence, each clinician must learn about human suffering's complexity.[9,10] Only with such awareness can the caregiver communicate effectively with patients and meet the needs of their personal circumstances and pain. Caregivers must also confront the prospects of their own deaths before they can fully help patients and their families face the end of life. Doing so will also help them optimize the beneficial effects of treatment along the way.

It is clear, however, that we can only assess individual healers in the context of the complex institutions and systems that connect them to patients. Recognition of this has spurred the development of covenants to define health care institutions' and organizations' relationship with patients and their social contract with the public.[11] Despite their undeniable value, these covenants do not seem to be restoring public trust in our health system or rebuilding health professionals' commitment to provide the best care. What is lacking to give these covenants force is a way to measure all the disparate elements that go into keeping them.

Although some would say that all the relevant elements cannot be measured, because some of them are inescapably diffuse and subjective, I believe the time has come to make the attempt. Such benchmarking is a way to rescue the health care enterprise from drowning in the riptides and storms of the marketplace. The measurements are also a way to help workaday health care professionals rediscover, reinstitute, and infuse into their organizations their own core professional values and interest in serving people. Finally, we must appreciate the findings of scholars, like organizational psychologist Michael Maccoby,[12] on how organizations and the people in them can change. Both can learn from current activities and thus may constantly move forward.

Because we become, or want to become, what we measure, I propose that we come up with a single number—a therapeutic index—by which the "healing whole" of a health care entity may be assessed over time. The Organizational Therapeutic Index (OTI) sets forth a measurement tool and model that an institution can adapt to its own needs (see appendix). It represents the first time an evaluative method has been developed to measure and track the elements of a successful therapeutic environment, in which mature healers from all the health professions interact with patients in a way that expresses the major American values of justice, mercy, hope, and autonomy. The OTI can serve learning organizations as a robust, flexible diagnostic and developmental tool.

Previous chapters have reviewed the characteristics that medical educators and health professionals have consistently aimed to exemplify and transmit. I believe that these characteristics—scientific competence, an understanding of suffering and death, good communication, respect for the placebo effect, commitment to three paradigms of service (prevention, curing, and caring), and loyalty to the patient and community—provide a basis for assessing the perform-ance of health care teams, health care institutions and organizations, and the entire American health care system.

In a previous attempt to analyze the foundational values of or-ganized health care systems, I identified four separate but interacting clusters of values: societal values; learning or university values; pro-fessional values; and business values. The societal values, already dis-cussed, are autonomy, justice, hope, and mercy.[13] The university or learning values are discovery, education (of the profession, public, and patients), and service. Professional values are the four Cs: competence, compassion, commitment, and collaboration. Business values include fair profit, effective distribution of goods and services, quality prod-ucts, and customer satisfaction.

Health Care in the American Grain

Our health care institutions and professionals, as I have empha-sized, are products of and are influenced by the history and traditions that form America's unique character. As we seek to understand where we are in health care, we would do well to reflect on what philosopher John McDermott, among others, refers to as "the Amer-ican grain," the core attributes that give substance, texture, and flavor to our particular culture and society.[14] These characteristics—most notably a lingering commitment to the frontier spirit, love of individual freedom, and devotion to technology, invention, and innovation—provide much of the substrate out of which American institutions have grown, including our health care systems and many of their individual pieces.[15, 16, 17, 18, 19] The development of the OTI model takes account of these unique underpinnings of Ameri-can society.

In their book *Habits of the Heart*, which I have already mentioned,

Robert Bellah and colleagues identify John Winthrop, the first governor of Massachusetts Bay Colony, as an example of an early American leader who placed overarching emphasis on the general welfare of the community.[20] Soon enough individuality, personified in the genius and personality of Benjamin Franklin, burst upon what was becoming our national consciousness. By the 1830s, Alexis de Tocqueville, the famous French observer of our experiment in democracy, described in exquisite detail in *Democracy in America* how the frontiersman, with his wife and children, his dog, an occasional neighbor, and his knife and gun, believed himself to be completely independent, relying on no social structure to sustain himself and his family. The intensity of this fierce independence, de Tocqueville worried, might ultimately prevent the new nation from meeting inevitable communal challenges. The tension between the ideals exemplified by Winthrop and Franklin can also be illustrated by comparing the concern with communal goals expressed both by the Constitution's stress on "promot[ing] the general welfare" and the Canadian national constitution's triad of "peace, order, and good government" with the Declaration of Independence's famous focus on "life, liberty, and the pursuit of happiness."

A related American hallmark is our passionate stand on freedom. According to historian Daniel Boorstin, as I have mentioned, our strong sense of freedom relies on rapid advances in technology. When he refers to America as "the Republic of Technology," he is doing more than just creating a catchy phrase. Boorstin explains that with the closing down of the nation's geographical frontiers, Americans have come to depend on the astounding flow of technological advances to prevent domination by any political demagogue or rigid belief system.[21] Today, expectation of the next technology sustains our sense of new space to explore and new freedom to conduct such exploration.

Our society might occasionally move forward too quickly with tantalizing new technologies. The late Paul G. Rogers, who over twenty-four years as a congressman from Florida spearheaded much of the country's most important public health, medical-scientific, and environmental legislation, brought this to my attention a few years ago when he recounted his reaction to a daylong conference on nanotechnology. He worried that unbridled optimism could boomerang on this promising new field, and that if we weren't careful to evaluate the risks along with the benefits, one early disaster could scare a skittish public from making necessary developmental investments.

Bellah et al. and Boorstin may or may not be right in all their interpretations. However, their observations of the American personality's celebration of individualism, independence, and technology ring true to me in general and in particular in the field of health care. The American approach to life made possible the independent physician free to work under professional guidelines and the fee-for-service paradigm. Today, the same forces contribute to the movement from a doctor-knows-best model toward a patient-centered model of health care.[22] In this newer model, patients participate, and may lead, in choosing diagnostic approaches and therapies, play an active role in the healing process, and no longer take the altruism of health care personnel for granted.

An increasingly important aspect of this trend occurs when patients take action on their own behalf, especially by using electronic communication to find and share information on diseases and treatment.[23] Such self-help and support networks[24] have grown dramatically since C. S. Bosk wrote of them in "The Transformation of the Therapeutic Relationship" in 1997. They highlight the American mentality, which is always seeking self-reliant venues to help solve individual and group problems, often without a clinician.

What Will the Twenty-first-Century American Health System Look Like?

A twenty-first-century American health system worthy of the country will provide access for every citizen to proven basic health care prevention, health promotion, and disease treatment. It will offer additional optional insurance plans to cover care not yet considered part of a basic and necessary package or where FDA-approved drugs or other technologies have not passed a rigorous evidence-based, cost-effectiveness standard. Its payment and incentive systems, along with an increasingly well-informed and activist population, will encourage patient-centered care and facilitate teamwork in delivering that care. Electronic medical records (with appropriate protections for patient confidentiality) will anchor cost-effective processes that enable society to afford health care for everyone.

This is America, and therefore we can expect many different models. We may have urban and rural models. There may be chronic disease-specific teams. There may be high-tech telemedicine and nursing models for isolated rural or elderly populations. Some patients may utilize more than one model and more than one (or even two different) health care teams. Such complexity will only increase the need for the electronic health record and the medical home.

If my recollection is correct, more than twenty years ago I heard Dr. Don Fredrickson—successively former head of the Institute of Medicine, the National Institutes of Health, and the Howard Hughes Medical Institute—talk about how wired and computerized health care had become in Denmark and Sweden. John Wennberg, Eliot Fisher, and their colleagues at the Dartmouth Atlas of Health Care have been generating data for decades showing how practices, costs, and outcomes differ from region to region and state to state across America. That there are differences in health care practices and costs among New England, Florida, Minnesota, and California shouldn't shock us any more than that there are similar differences among Portugal, England, Italy, Norway, and Germany. In making international comparisons, it may be useful to recall that France is about the size of Texas and Europe approximates the size of the United States. What is crucial is that such studies provoke the right questions, which with the proper sociopolitical will can lead America to a more uniform and equitable distribution of the best and most cost-effective health care.

The Organizational Therapeutic Index: We Are What We Measure

This sample of my proposal for evaluative measures of twenty-first-century health care organizations and clinical practices could be diagrammed as starting from a basic value, moving to a specific goal, then to guideposts, and finally to quantifiable benchmarks for the structure, process, and outcomes of care. Let's take as an example one of our four basic values: autonomy. That value would lead us to a goal of achieving patient autonomy. That goal might in turn suggest that guideposts in achieving this goal should begin with properly designed patient and family satisfaction surveys. These surveys in turn might suggest such benchmarks as the presence and proper utilization of electronic medical records, bar-coding of patient medications, and additional targeted surveys from patients, caregivers, and administrators. Each benchmark can be weighted to provide a basis for year-over-year comparison of an institution's or organization's progress in supporting patient autonomy.

The same process can be followed to designate institutional goals and relevant quantifiable benchmarks for justice, mercy, and hope. In the detailed Organizational Therapeutic Index I have devised, I have included as goals, categorized under one of the four basic values, each of the six "healer's" characteristics listed earlier: scientific competence;

understanding suffering and death; ability to communicate; knowledge of the placebo effect; expanding roles in three paradigms of care; commitment and loyalty to the patient and public. As with the simplified version above of translating the value autonomy into specific benchmarks, one can select from a variety of existing and often commonly used standards to assess institutional and individual health care performance. Then it is a matter of judgment how much weight each should have in the final index number for a particular health care institution or clinical practice.

An academic health center's university hospital and clinics might weight scientific competence as 60 percent of the final grade, but it could just as easily be 40 or 85 percent. Different practice settings, ranging from a solo primary care or specialty practice to a large multipractitioner specialty practice or a multihospital system, would naturally have different weightings for each measure. If an obstetrical practice were judging the relative importance of how they handled suffering and death, they should want to do the best they could in the area, but it would not constitute as big a piece of the pie as if their organization were a hospice. Both might score perfectly in their handling of suffering and death, but for one of them the measure might represent only 5 percent of their total OTI, whereas for the other it might represent 75 percent.

The strength and beauty of this sort of model are precisely that it can be customized for each institution. In fact, it is impossible to develop one model for every setting. Effective health care measurement requires a collaborative institutional effort to develop goals, select the therapeutic elements that will fulfill the goals, identify the specific instruments that can provide data for benchmarking each element, ascribe weights to the different components, and develop infrastructure to accomplish the job. An overarching committee representing all parts of the institution should meet and monitor progress during the year and set priorities for improvement for each subsequent year. The process would not always be easy, but one can envision first-class health professionals and administrators engaging in it with enthusiasm, especially if they could see tangible progress.

The sample model detailed in the appendix is for the most complex institutions and organizations; simpler models may be sufficient for others. But in any case I hope the model shows that it is indeed possible to measure performance in providing justice, compassion, hope, and autonomy in health care.

One final caveat. It is all well and good to speak about measuring our performance in terms of the noblest human aspirations, but it would be folly to do so without recognizing the great extent to which the effort to care for the sick and disabled, prevent disease, and promote healthy living has been engulfed by monetary interests and concerns. I will leave it up to others to debate whether mercy can turn a profit, and if so, how much! However, I have found it enlightening to follow corporate guru Jim Collins and his team through their researches on how successful corporations function and are led. In his hugely influential and impressive book *Good to Great*, Collins addresses one central idea: the hedgehog concept. He draws three intersecting circles to measure a company's financial performance over a period of fifteen years in comparison with others in the Fortune 500. The three circles represent what the company does best, what it is most passionate about, and how it makes money. The best companies exemplify the hedgehog concept by focusing predominantly on the overlap between the three.

Collins has recently published an essay-sized booklet entitled *Good to Great in the Social Sectors: Why Business Thinking Is Not the Answer*. After studying a series of not-for-profit organizations, he and his team drew a new set of three intersecting circles. Two circles were familiar from his books on business companies: what the organization does best and what the organization is most passionate about. The third circle did not represent financial revenues and profits, but success in "branding"; that is, the enterprise's ability to identify and attract the people and sectors it seeks to serve.

In Collins's analysis, social sector excellence requires measuring success without business metrics, using different leadership skills, rethinking the economic engine minus the profit motive, and building momentum by building the brand. Therefore, he says, "We need to reject the naïve imposition of the language of business on the social sectors, and instead jointly embrace a language of greatness."[25]

Twenty-first-century American health care is of course big business and big politics. Private enterprise intertwines inextricably with public and not-for-profit megaliths. Our health professional stars do very well financially, and the social status of the health professions generally is quite high and getting higher. Health care company executives and not-for-profit and public health managers and leaders are no less competent or less well compensated than their counterparts in other major national industries. The science and technology base continues to explode, preparing the way for future diagnostic, therapeutic, and sustaining tools. The federal government plays a major role, with proven capabilities in many vast health care enterprises from Medicare to Medicaid, SCHIP, and the Veterans Administration.

Economic and political forces have converged around a push for positive change in our nation's health status and for the elimination of inequitable health care distribution and major health disparities in various population groups. Some major changes in health care seem likely in the near future, the first steps in what will undoubtedly be an ongoing process of large-scale economic negotiation and political compromise.

But human beings receive health care one at a time. Individuals care about the values that drive their lives, such as hope for the future, justice, mercy, and personal autonomy. How can our society harness those values and express them through its health care services, and how can individuals find out how health professionals and organizations are living up to those values? As I hope the reader will find in the appendix describing the Organizational Therapeutic Index, there is good evidence that even the most complex organizations can measure their effectiveness, efficiency, and capacity to live up to the highest of our American values.

The ultimate challenge of the years ahead is putting it all together in each individual's life. The ability to meet this challenge—that patients and their surrogates serve as board chairs of their individual health care companies—is now within our reach. Growing numbers of increasingly sophisticated patients will advocate for this model within the national health care dialogue. Indeed, they are already beginning to do so, and I believe it is in these terms that society can embrace a new language of greatness in health care. Each of us will eventually be able to direct our own virtual health care company, assisted by our chosen professional counselors and empowered by a computer and Web-based communication and data systems.

The personal health care company will not march at government command! It will be as individual an enterprise as each person's exercise of the rights to life, liberty, and the pursuit of happiness. Such may be, after all, the twenty-first-century American way to a healthier society.

Appendix

The Organizational Therapeutic Index Model

Adapting the Organizational Therapeutic Index (OTI) to the needs of a health care institution or practice and its people should begin with a broad-based committee of administrators, health care professionals, staff, and patients. In the case of institutions, representatives from both the patient and local communities should play important, ongoing roles. This approach encourages both lay and professional stakeholders to take ownership of the effort to improve performance based upon shared clinical values and self-determined institutional or organizational goals. The CEO of the institution, in turn, should create positive incentives to encourage staff to improve therapeutic performance scores. The strongest signal would be for the CEO to chair the OTI committee; at the least it should report directly to the CEO.

I have utilized eleven elements to determine the OTI, in part so that a group or organization can dedicate one month a year to a special focus on each element. That leaves the twelfth month available for an overall review of the scores achieved and an analysis of the weaknesses discovered. The OTI could of course have more or fewer elements, but no matter how it is structured, there should be an institutionwide OTI evaluation at least once a year.

Methodology

A logical approach to apportioning committee tasks would be to assign a subcommittee to each therapeutic element being measured, and to have this group determine which instruments can, over time, yield a good measurement of progress in that area. The committee can then conduct the review itself, or assign this task to other qualified people.

Three tasks, however, logically fall under the province of the full OTI committee. The first is to decide on the therapeutic elements to be evaluated and set the goals for each element. One goal for "understanding suffering and pain, death and dying," for example, would be to prevent unnecessary acute exacerbations or manifestations of chronic underlying diseases, such as diabetes or asthma.

The second task is to assign a maximum score to the OTI. This single number represents what the institution has determined possible in terms of the measure it has chosen. In my illustrative model the score is 100.

The third task for the committee is assigning maximum scores for each element in keeping with the institution's mission. For example, depending on the institution's patient-care purposes, the committee might weight the score for scientific and technical competency at anywhere from 40 to 80 percent of the total possible OTI score.

The relevant subcommittee can then step in to determine which instruments can best measure a particular element over time. The organization may have to devote resources to customize or develop such instruments. The subcommittee should also determine the weight of each measurement chosen for benchmarking. Because a particular measurement may apply more than once in a single OTI, its weight should vary depending on the element being assessed.

Making the OTI an important factor in institutional morale and performance in today's environment of constant flux means keeping data-gathering measures up to date as the years roll on. To this end, it is important to analyze the number of times each evaluative measure is used and also compile the total number of points that each measure can earn.

The OTI deploys 35 basic measures to evaluate 109 indicators of the therapeutic institution. Many measurement instruments have multiple uses. Patient surveys, for example, are important for measuring performance in virtually every element, whereas surveys of family members, nurses, and physicians are important for evaluating two-thirds of the elements. Although all measures must be up to date, the questions in these survey instruments in particular should be specifically tailored to each therapeutic element.

Furthermore, how much each measure contributes to an entity's OTI depends on what kind of health care institution or practice it is. The most influential measures in the sample OTI are hospital readmission rates for certain chronic diseases (2e); the pain management protocol (4a); care for the terminally ill (4b); patient-satisfaction, nurse-satisfaction, and physician-satisfaction surveys (5a, 5c, 5d, respectively); and "magnet hospital" status (6c).

The Elements That Heal

Many of the selected instruments, particularly for scientific and technical competence, are already used by accrediting and other organizations, including health care entities. What is different about their use in the OTI is their application to developing, measuring, and sustaining an organizational culture of healing.

PUTTING SCIENTIFIC AND TECHNICAL COMPETENCE FIRST

The most important therapeutic element to measure in any health care entity is scientific and technical competence. Only a few decades ago, a hospital's medical staff could attest to the qualifications of new staff by checking applicants' credentials and establishing appropriate mechanisms to follow various areas of practice. The organization's administrative arm, in turn, was responsible for the ongoing surveillance of professional competence. Now, even with the Joint Commission on the Accreditation of Health Care Organizations (JCAHO) sharpening its focus on the quality of clinical care, evaluating a health care institution's competence is becoming increasingly complex. I selected the cluster of measures in table 1 to evaluate the scientific and technical competence at the health care institution I have in mind. To each of these twenty-four measures, I have assigned a value ranging from 1.0 to 3.0, seeking to achieve a maximum of 60 points for the entire therapeutic element.

UNDERSTANDING PAIN AND SUFFERING, DEATH, AND DYING

Expert clinicians understand that clinically relevant suffering and pain range from the mental anguish of dealing with the intractable pain of certain stages of serious disease to coping with a potentially life-shortening situation. This connection is why experts on the humane treatment of the dying insist that excellent palliative care must be available to most patients. From the myriad possible examples illustrating the importance of this element, let me use only one: the treatment of people with asthma and chronic obstructive pulmonary disease (COPD). In both groups of patients, the occurrence of acute obstructive exacerbations submits the patient to frightening shortness of breath and a life-threatening situation. We now know how to reduce the frequency of such acute episodes and thereby considerably reduce patient suffering. This treatment, however, is usually nonreimbursable. Ironically, a metric that sets up effective procedures for these patients and reduces their rate of annual hospitalization will call attention to a perverse financial incentive for the institution, while rewarding the courage to do right by the patient. For my hypothetical health care institution, the nine measures used to evaluate this element appear in table 2. Each measure receives 0.25 to 3.0 points for a maximum of 12 points.

APPRECIATING THE PLACEBO EFFECT

The placebo effect, in its strictest definition, refers to unexplained results associated with the application of a drug, procedure, or other medical intervention. It does not mean fooling patients by giving them sugar pills and encouraging them to believe in their curative effectiveness. It can be considered when a patient has improved for no obvious reason. This effect is relevant to efforts to enhance the therapeutic effectiveness of an entire hospital, clinic, or health care system. Whether or not one is comfortable with the use of the placebo terminology, the bottom line is that better patient outcomes are likely to happen if a relationship of trust is established across an entire organization. All those working in the organization need to understand their role in building trust not only with patients but also with their families. Furthermore, all caregivers have to deliver the same or similar messages to the patient regarding the patient's health status, future prospects, and care. In table 3, the nine evaluative instruments for appreciating the placebo effect range from 0.25 to 2.0 points in value for a total of 4.0 points.

EXPANDING HEALTH CARE ROLES AND RESPONSIBILITIES

The aging of the population is leading us to better ways to keep people, elderly or not, functioning outside of institutions as long as possible. At the same time, all sectors of the health care enterprise are coming to understand that issues of cost, quality, and access to health care make it essential for each health care system component to think in terms of its particular role and responsibilities across the full range of essential services. The organization's OTI, therefore, should reflect a commitment to set up and maintain a successful interface, after discharge, with the frail elderly and with patients who have serious chronic conditions. The OTI, for example, should include appropriate measures of the organization's expanded effort in health promotion and disease prevention (HPDP), which has become a national priority. At one end of the discharge spectrum are vaccines to be administered and health-promoting behaviors to be reinforced. At the other end are the many behavior and support mechanisms and developments in advanced technologies that lead to more efficient coping strategies, especially for incurable chronic diseases. There are also programs that prevent exacerbations and clinical relapses or offer systemic care. Table 4 lists ten measures, ranging from 0.1 to 0.5 of a point in value, and adding up to 3 points, giving but one example of how a large institution can evaluate its handling of expanded responsibilities.

COMMUNICATING DIGNITY AND RESPECT

In today's health care scene, there are times and places where the patient, already vulnerable to losing basic human dignity and feeling disrespected, can become frightened or anxious at the slightest oversight or misstep. A classic example occurs when someone is wheeled down to the X-ray department on a gurney—all too reminiscent of how corpses are removed from the ward and travel to the morgue or autopsy room—at what seems like blinding speed, only to be left in a hallway, often a little cold and uncovered, for an uncertain period of time, without an apparent handoff to another responsible individual. Five instruments that can measure respect for the patient appear in table 5, totaling 6 points. The instruments receive from 0.5 to 2.0 points.

DEMONSTRATING ORGANIZATIONAL LOYALTY TO PATIENTS:

How much do we really care about the ongoing well-being of our patients? How do we best show our concern for them across the entire institution? These kinds of questions get to the heart of the quality and endurance of any relationship between patients and those who render their health care. The better and more firmly rooted this relationship, the greater the trust between the professional caregiver and the recipient of care. It is reasonable to assume that the combination of high levels of trust and professional and technical skill will produce the best possible clinical outcomes. Table 6 lists nine instruments for evaluating organization-to-patient loyalty in our model. Each receives 0.5 to 1.0 point for a maximum score of 5 points.

MAKING THE PATIENT PART OF THE HEALTH CARE TEAM

Along with other elements of the American psyche, individualism continues to assert itself in our health care system. It is the individual who typically chooses the clinician, the clinical organization, and the kind of health insurance to have or whether to have insurance at all. It is the individual who wants to preserve the privacy of his or her hospital record as much and as long as possible. Any therapeutic patient-centered organization must seek to understand the nature and effectiveness of the patient's role in determining or influencing the care to be received. Even a patient not yet fully empowered as the chair of a personal health care board has earned full rights to membership on the clinical team. The five different measures in table 7, each weighing in at from 0.25 to 1.0 point and totaling 2 points, are examples of the instruments a health care institution can use to assess the extent and quality of patients' participation on their health care teams.

Emphasizing Teamwork and Collaboration

Teamwork is an important marker of an organization's therapeutic effectiveness. Demand for team care grows daily, and evidence continues to mount that good teamwork is essential to providing multiprofessional care and also to improving certain specifics of care; for example, the error rate in hospital performance or the number of hospital-acquired infections. Devising specific measures to assess teamwork in health care is a difficult undertaking, because a number of teams may be working simultaneously for the same patient. Obviously, some teams will do better than others, and one team may be doing better at one moment than it has done in the past or will do in the future. Such variations must be taken into account. Table 8 includes seven measures of teamwork and collaboration, each receiving 0.1 to 1.0 point for a possible total of 3 points. Staff turnover rates and exit interviews appear for the first time. I include them because I believe that institutions with the strongest team ethos generally have the lowest workforce turnover rates and the highest overall employee satisfaction.

Taking the Environment into Account

Large health care institutions frequently remodel their older facilities or build entirely new ones. These efforts should increasingly be oriented toward creating healthy, pleasing, energy-efficient, cost-effective, and environmentally sustainable structures. We are learning much about the positive impact of a physical environment that is calming, offers a view of the outdoors, and provides a friendly setting for patients and their families. Health care institutions should not, even out of ignorance, be in the business of building and maintaining "sick" buildings. Rather, we must seek to build the healthiest of buildings that can approach energy sustainability. The atmosphere created by the behavior of staff and administration also constitutes part of the therapeutic environment. This more subtle environmental effect, as reflected in various support activities and other explicit efforts to create a service culture, also deserves careful assessment. The twelve instruments suggested for measuring this element of health care performance appear in table 9. Their weighted values range from 0.1 to 0.5 of a point for a total of 2.0 points.

Affirming Cultural Sensitivity and Workforce Diversity

Most health care organizations have to take into account the huge increase in immigration from countries all over the globe, which has in turn stretched available health care resources. One result is that in many places, communication with non-English-speaking patients threatens to be severely restricted, deepening deficits in cultural understanding. Table 10 lists two evaluative markers, totaling 1.5 points, that can measure and follow the sensitivity of an institution to an evolving, racially and ethnically diverse constituency. For this element especially, the huge variance in demographic makeup from locale to locale compels every institution to map its own plan for cultural sensitivity and workforce diversity.

Working with the Community

Community citizenship has become an important part of forward-looking organizations throughout the public service and business sectors. Certainly health care organizations, large and small, have always been close to the heart of their communities. This has been even more true since 9/11 and the growing awareness of the fragility of our emergency-preparedness systems at local, regional, and national levels. One large, not-for-profit health care enterprise has established a vice president for community service, funding the activity by tying the expenditure budget to what its taxes would have been had it been a for-profit entity. Such an approach could be used for public health and some bioterrorism procedures and functions. As each organization assesses its community's needs and its potential to respond to some of those needs, it will invariably develop a to-do list. The list may range from overall economic impact (the institution is usually one of the largest employers in the community) to specific public education efforts related to science and health to specific activities aimed at underserved or needy populations. Table 11 assesses working with the community on the basis of nine measures, ranging from 0.05 to 0.3 of a point, for a total of 1.45 points.

The Strength of the OTI

The OTI should serve as an organizational self-study tool, with staff, patients, and other stakeholders selecting existing data and tailoring surveys and focus groups to reflect the elements of a culture of healing. It is not a tool for comparing one institution with another, because each may decide to use different elements or to weight the same elements differently. Instead, the OTI facilitates self-comparison and growth over the years. Obviously, one size will not fit all, and certainly this sample OTI, which was built with a large hospital or health system in mind, is not appropriate for smaller clinical groups serving smaller populations of patients. However, it would not be difficult for such groups to customize their own OTI. The important thing is to include our highest aspirations and ideals for civilized health care into an evaluative tool we can use. Then, day by day, we will be able to look around the health care playing field and ensure that we are living up to our oaths, covenants, and hopes.

Table 1. Sample OTI Measures for Scientific and Technical Competence

Measures by Category	Maximum Points
1. Risk-adjusted mortality, total category	8.00
a. Surgical mortality rate	2.00
b. Medical mortality rate	2.00
c. Anesthesia mortality rate	2.00
d. Cardiac mortality rate	1.00
e. Cancer mortality rate	1.00
2. JCAHO and other standard criteria, total category	15.00
a. Sentinel events: number reported	3.00
b. Overall error rate: percentage with damage, causing fatality, drug related	3.00
c. Number of reports on possible errors or near misses	3.00
d. Rate of hospital-acquired infections	3.00
e. Hospital readmission rates, especially for chronic diseases	3.00
3. Paperless environment, total category	12.00
a. Electronic order entry	3.00
b. Electronic records and restricted accessibility	3.00
c. Bar-coding for pharmaceutical administration	3.00
d. Electronic, automatic patient follow-up and reminder postdischarge	3.00
4. Evidence-based protocols, total category	10.00
a. Pain management	3.00
b. Care for terminally ill, including hospice care transfer	2.00
c. Weekly discharge rounds, reviews	3.00
d. Cancer, BP, diabetes and complications screening; compliance data	2.00

Measures by Category	Maximum Points
5. Surveys and focus groups, total category	11.00
a. Patient satisfaction: secure/confident in care received	3.00
b. Nurse satisfaction and quality-of-care survey: secure in care given	3.00
c. MD satisfaction and quality-of-care survey: secure in care given	3.00
d. Community MD and nurse reviews of care quality in entity reviewed	2.00
6. Administrative processes and policies, total category	4.00
a. Magnet hospital status for excellence in nursing	3.00
b. Doulas for OB/GYN service; social services	1.00
TOTAL	**60.00**

Table 2. Sample OTI Measures for Understanding of Pain and Suffering, Death and Dying

Measures by Category	Maximum Points
1. Selected JCAHO and other standard criteria, total category	0.25
a. Hospital readmission rates for chronic diseases such as diabetes, heart disease, hypertension, asthma	0.25
2. Paperless environment, total category	0.50
a. Bar-coding for pharmaceutical administration	0.25
b. Electronic, automatic patient follow-up postdischarge	0.25
3. Evidence-based protocols, total category	5.25
a. Pain management	3.00
b. Care for terminally ill, including hospice care transfer	2.00
c. Cancer screening tests; BP screening; diabetes and complications screening; data in compliance with standard practices	0.25
4. Surveys and focus groups, total category	2.00
a. Patient satisfaction: secure and confident in care received	1.00
b. Family communication and follow-through	1.00

Measures by Category	Maximum Points
5. Administrative processes and policies, total category	4.00
a. Magnet hospital status for excellence in nursing	1.00
b. Two-way communication; printout of individual patient's next-day schedule ready each night; electronic/Internet programs	0.50
c. Number of hospital/provider committees that include patients	0.50
d. Percentage of patient rooms with windows	0.50
e. Doulas for OB/GYN service; social services	0.50
f. Cultural sensitivity: number of interpreters available/number of foreign languages spoken by patients; workforce diversity measures	0.50
g. Staff education programs on pain, suffering, death and dying	0.50
TOTAL	**12.00**

Table 3. Sample OTI Measures for Appreciating the Placebo Effect

Measures by Category	Maximum Points
1. Evidence-based protocols, total category	0.20
a. Pain management	0.20
2. Surveys and focus groups, total category	0.30
a. Patient satisfaction: secure and confident in care received	0.20
b. Family communication and follow-through	0.10
3. Administrative processes and policies, total category	3.50
a. Magnet hospital status for excellence in nursing	1.00
b. Two-way communication; daily individual patient schedule printout available the night before; electronic/Internet programs	1.00
c. Percentage of patient rooms with windows	0.50
d. Cultural sensitivity: number of available interpreters/number of foreign languages spoken by patients; workforce diversity measures	0.25
e. Staff education programs on building patient trust, etc.	0.25
f. Disclosure at regular intervals (annually or more frequently) of performance progress and results of OTI, broken down by therapeutic element, demonstrating organization's interest in being held accountable	0.50
TOTAL	**4.00**

Table 4. Sample OTI Measures for
Expanding Health Care Roles and Responsibilities

Measures by Category	Maximum Points
1. Selected JCHA and other standard criteria, total category	0.50
a. Hospital readmission rates, especially for chronic diseases such as diabetes, heart disease, hypertension, asthma	0.50
2. Paperless environment, total category	0.20
a. Electronic, automatic patient follow-up and reminder postdischarge	0.20
3. Evidence-based protocols, total category	0.80
a. Weekly discharge rounds, reviews	0.30
b. Cancer screening tests; BP, diabetes and complications screening; data in compliance with standard practices	0.50
4. Surveys and focus groups, total category	0.30
a. Patient satisfaction: secure and confident in care received	0.10
b. Family communication and follow-through	0.10
c. MD satisfaction and quality-of-care survey: secure and confident in the care they give	0.10
5. Administrative processes and policies, total category	1.20
a. Annual plan and director for community service in place	0.50
b. Doulas for OB/GYN service; social services	0.20
c. Disclosure at regular intervals of progress/results of OTI, etc.	0.50
TOTAL	**3.00**

Table 5. Sample OTI Measures for
Communicating Dignity and Respect

Measures by Category	Maximum Points
1. Surveys and focus groups, total category	2.50
a. Patient satisfaction: secure and confident in care received	2.00
b. Family communication and follow-through	0.50
2. Administrative processes and policies, total category	3.50
a. Two-way communication; daily individual patient next-day	

schedule printout distributed each night; electronic/Internet
   programs   1.50
b. Cultural sensitivity: number of interpreters on hand/number of
   foreign languages spoken by patients; workforce diversity
   measures   1.50
c. Staff educational programs on building patient trust and
   confidence   0.50

TOTAL   **6.00**

Table 6. Sample OTI Measures for Demonstrating Organizational Loyalty to Patients

Measures by Category	Maximum Points
1. Surveys and focus groups, total category	3.00
a. Patient satisfaction: secure and confident in care received	1.00
b. Family communication and follow-through	0.50
c. Nurse satisfaction and quality-of-care survey: secure/ confident in their care	0.50
d. MD satisfaction and quality-of-care survey: secure/ confident in their care	0.50
e. Community MD and nurse views of care at this health care entity	0.50
2. Administrative processes and policies, total categories	2.00
a. Two-way communication, etc. (as detailed in table 5, item 2a)	0.50
b. Percentage of patient rooms with windows	0.50
c. Cultural sensitivity: etc. (as detailed in table 5, item 2b)	0.50
d. Staff educational programs on building patient trust and confidence	0.50
TOTAL	**5.00**

Table 7. Sample OTI Measures for Making the Patient Part of the Health Care Team

Measures by Category	Maximum Points
1. Surveys and focus groups, total category	1.00
a. Patient satisfaction: secure and confident in care received	0.25

b. Family communication and follow-through	0.25
c. Nurse satisfaction and quality of care survey: confidence in care	0.25
d. MD satisfaction and quality of care survey: confidence in care	0.25
2. Administrative processes and policies, total category	1.00
a. Two-way communication, etc. (as detailed in table 5, item 2a)	1.00
TOTAL	**2.00**

Table 8. Sample OTI Measures for Teamwork and Collaboration

Measures by Category	Maximum Points
1. Selected JCAHO and other standard criteria, total category	0.50
a. Overall error rate: percentage causing patient damage, percentage contributing to death, percentage of all errors that are pharmacological or drug related	0.20
b. Rate of hospital-acquired infections	0.10
c. Hospital readmission rates, especially for chronic diseases such as diabetes, heart disease, hypertension, and asthma	0.20
2. Surveys and focus groups, total category	2.40
a. Patient satisfaction: secure and confident in care received	1.00
b. Nurse satisfaction and quality-of-care survey: confidence in care they give	0.70
c. MD satisfaction and quality-of-care survey: confidence in care they give	0.70
3. Administrative processes and policies, total category	0.10
a. Staff turnover rates; nurse turnover rates; employee satisfaction, exit interview summaries	0.10
TOTAL	**3.00**

Table 9. Sample OTI Measures for
Taking the Environment into Account

Measures by Category	Maximum Points
1. Surveys and focus groups, total category	0.60
a. Patient satisfaction: secure and confident in care received	0.10
b. Family communication and follow-through	0.10
c. Nurse satisfaction and quality of care survey: confidence in care given	0.20
d. MD satisfaction and quality of care survey: confidence in care given	0.10
e. Community survey regarding reputation of health care entity	0.10
2. Administrative processes and policies, total category	1.40
a. Evidence of CEO leadership in quality/safety issues	0.20
b. Percentage of patient rooms with windows	0.20
c. Staff turnover and nurse turnover rates, employee satisfaction; exit interview summaries	0.10
d. Doulas for OB/GYN service; social services	0.10
e. Cultural sensitivity: number of interpreters/number of languages of patients; workforce diversity measures	0.10
f. Staff educational programs regarding terminal care, building patient trust, system safety, sustainable "green" and healthy buildings/environments	0.50
g. Disclosure at regular intervals of performance progress of OTI progress and results, broken down by individual elements	0.20
TOTAL	**2.00**

Table 10. Sample OTI Measures for Affirming
Cultural Sensitivity and Workforce Diversity

Measures by Category	Maximum Points
1. Administrative processes and policies, total category	1.50
a. Cultural sensitivity: number of interpreters/number of languages spoken by patients; workforce diversity measures; staff and patient satisfaction surveys	1.00
b. Staff educational programs on relevant diversity/cultural issues	0.50
TOTAL	**1.50**

Table 11. Sample OTI Measures for Working with the Community

Measures by Category	Maximum Points
1. Surveys and focus groups, total category	0.35
a. Patient satisfaction with care	0.10
b. Family communication and follow-through	0.05
c. Nurse satisfaction/confidence in care given	0.05
d. MD satisfaction/confidence in care given	0.05
e. Community MD and nurse opinion of health care entity regarding care given	0.15
2. Administrative processes and policies, total category	1.10
a. Annual plan and director for community service in place	0.50
b. Cultural sensitivity: interpreters, languages and workforce diversity	0.10
c. Staff educational programs on community impact issues	0.30
d. Annual report on community program results/contributions	0.20
TOTAL	**1.50**

Notes

Chapter 1: A Physician's Lessons from Being a Patient

1. Leston Havens, *Making Contact: Uses of Language in Psychotherapy* (Harvard University Press: Cambridge, 1986).

2. Roger J. Bulger, *The Quest for Mercy* (Cardin-Jennings: Charlottesville, 1998), 21.

3. John C. Vander Woude, "The Care-giver as a Patient" in *The Doctor as a Person* (Charles C. Thomas: Springfield, IL, 1988), 188–195.

4. Fitzhugh Mullan, *Vital Signs: A Young Doctor's Struggle with Cancer* (Farrar, Straus & Giroux: New York, 1975), 31.

5. Jennifer Hecht, *The Happiness Myth* (HarperCollins: New York, 2007).

6. Roger J. Bulger, "When Doctors Are Patients: Is There Such a Thing as Posttraumatic Bliss?," *Medscape Journal of Medicine* 10 (2008): 8.

7. Randy Pausch,, *The Last Lecture* (Hyperion: New York, 2008).

8. Viktor E. Frankl, *Man's Search for Meaning* (Beacon Press: Boston, 1959).

9. Viktor E. Frankl, *Man's Search for Ultimate Meaning* (Beacon Press: Boston, 1997).

10. David Rieff, *Swimming in a Sea of Death* (Simon & Shuster: New York, 2008).

11. E. B. White, *Here Is New York* (Little Bookroom: New York, 1999).

12. Richard Cohen, *Strong at the Broken Places* (HarperCollins: New York, 2008).

Chapter 2: Healing with Technology and with Words, Art, and the Senses

1. This discussion of language in medicine and the Hippocratic approach is taken in part from a lecture I delivered in Chicago at the University of Illinois Centennial Celebration, June 4, 1992, "Emerging Unities of the Twenty-first Century: Service as Secular Sacrament, Emotional Neutrality, and the Power of the Therapeutic Word."

2. Scott Stossel, "Still Crazy After All These Years: A History and Analysis of Psychotherapy from Freud's Couch to the Present," *New York Times Book Review*, Dec. 28, 2008, 16–17.

3. Norman Cousins, *Anatomy of an Illness* (Bantam Books: New York, 1979).

4. John Kennell, Marshall Klaus, Susan McGrath, Steven, Robertson, and Clark Hinkley, "Continuous Emotional Support During Labor in a U.S. Hospital," *Journal of the American Medical Association* 265 (1991): 2197–2201.

5. Cousins, *Anatomy of an Illness*.

6. Ibid.

7. Havens, *Making Contact*.

8. Cousins, *Anatomy of an Illness*.

9. Bernie S. Siegel, *Love, Medicine, and Miracles* (Harper & Row: New York, 1986).

10. Lewis Thomas, "House Calls" in *On Doctoring* (Simon & Schuster: New York, 1986).

11. Charles Fletcher and Paul Freeling, *Talking and Listening to Patients: A Modern Approach* (Nuffield Provincial Hospitals Trust, London, 1988).

12. Ibid.

13. Judee K. Burgoon, Michael Pfau, Roxanne Parrott, Thomas Birk, Ray Coker, and Michael Burgoon, "Relational Communication, Satisfaction, Compliance-gaining Strategies, and Compliance in Communication between Physicians and Patients," *Communication Monographs* 54 (1987): 307–324.

14. Philip A. Tumulty, "What Is a Clinician and What Does He Do?" in *On Doctoring* (Simon & Shuster: New York, 1986).

15. Dana Atchley, "Patient-Physician Communication" in *On Doctoring* (Simon & Shuster: New York, 1986).

16. George L. Engel, "How Much Longer Must Medicine's Science Be Bound by a Seventeenth Century World View?" in *The Task of Medicine* (Henry J. Kaiser Foundation: Menlo Park, 1988).

17. Max Delbruck, *Mind from Matter? An Essay on Evolutionary Epistemology* (Blackwell Scientific Publications: Palo Alto, 1986).

18. Amy Chua, *Day of Empire: How Hyperpowers Rise to Global Dominance—and Why They Fall*, (Doubleday: New York, 2007).

19. Daniel J. Boorstin, *Hidden History* (Harper & Row: New York, 1987).

20. Robert N. Bellah, Richard Madsen, William M. Sullivan, and Ann Swidler, *Habits of the Heart* (Harper & Row: New York, 1985).

21. Frankl, *Man's Search for Meaning*.

22. Dennis Ford, *The Search for Meaning: A Short History* (University of California. Press: Berkeley, 2007).

23. Susan Neiman, *Moral Clarity: A Guide for Grown-up Idealists* (Harcourt: New York, 2008).

24. John J. McDermott, "The Inevitability of Our Own Death" in *Streams of Experience: Reflections on the History and Philosophy of American Culture* (University of Massachusetts Press: Amherst, 1986), 168.

25. Robert Burton, *On Being Certain: Believing You Are Right, Even When You're Not* (St. Martin's Press: New York, 2008).

26. Fletcher and Freeling, *Talking and Listening to Patients*. (Nuffield Trust, London, 1989)

27. R. J. Bulger, "The Humanities and the Arts" in *In Search of the Modern Hippocrates* (University of Iowa Press: Iowa City, 1987).

28. "The Art of Healing," *Modern Health Care* (Dec. 21/28, 1992): 56.

29. Ibid.

30. R. S. Ulrich, "View through a Window May Influence Recovery from Surgery," *Science* 224, April 1984, 420–421.

31. Guido Majno, "The Lost Secret of Ancient Medicine," *In Search of the Modern Hippocrates* (University of Iowa Press: Iowa City, 1987).

32. John Beaulieu, *Music and Sound in the Healing Arts* (Station Hill Press: Barrytown, NY, 1987).

33. These associations are the National Association for Music Therapy in Washington, DC, and the American Association for Music Therapy in Springfield, New Jersey.

Chapter 3: Self-Healing, Our Internal Pharmacy, and the Placebo Effect

1. As quoted by F. J. Ingelfinger in "Medicine: Meritorious or Meretricious?" *Science* 200, May 1978, 942.

2. A. K. Shapiro, "Factors Contributing to the Placebo Effect: Their Implications for Psychotherapy," *American Journal of Psychotherapy* 18 (1961): 73.

3. H. Benson and D. P. McCallie, "Angina Pectoris and the Placebo Effect," *New England Journal of Medicine* 300 (1979): 1424.

4. R. G. Gallimore and J. L. Turner, "Contemporary Studies of Placebo Phenomena," *Psychopharmacology in the Practice of Medicine* (Appleton-Century-Crofts: New York, 1977), 47.

5. S. Wolf, "Effects of Suggestion and Conditioning on the Action of Chemical Agents in Human Subjects: The Pharmacology of Placebos," *Journal of Clinical Investigation* 29 (1950): 100.

6. Gallimore and Turner, "Contemporary Studies of Placebo Phenomena."

7. Herbert Benson and Mark D. Epstein, "The Placebo Effect: A Neglected Asset in the Care of Patients," *Journal of the American Medical Association* 232 (1975): 1225.

8. A. K. Shapiro, "Placebo Effects in Psychotherapy and Psychoanalysis," *Journal of Clinical Pharmacology* 10 (1970): 73.

9. J. A. Turner, R. A. Deyo, J. D. Loeser, M. Von Korff, and W. E. Fordyce, "The Importance of Placebo in Pain Treatment and Research," *Journal of the American Medical Association* 271 (1994): 1609–1614.

10. W. B. Cannon, "Voodoo Death," *American Anthropologist* 44 (April–June 1942): 169.

11. G. L. Engel, "Sudden and Rapid Death during Psychological Stress: Folklore or Folk Wisdom?" *Annals of Internal Medicine* 74 (1971): 711.

12. G. W. Milton, 1973. "Self-willed Death or the Bone-pointing Syndrome," *Lancet* 1 (1973): 1435.

13. S. Wolf, "Effects of Suggestion and Conditioning on the Action of Chemical Agents in Human Subjects, *The Journal of Clinical Investigations* 29 (January, 1950): 100-109."

14. S. Wolf and M. A. Pinsky, "Effects of Placebo Administration and Occurrence of Toxic Reactions," *Journal of the American Medical Association* 155 (1954): 339.

15. Institute of Medicine, National Academy of Sciences, *Behavioral Influences*

on the Endocrine and Immune Systems (National Academy Press: Washington, DC, 1989).

16. G. K. Kiecolt-Glaser and R. Glaser, "Psychological Influences on Immunity." *Immunity* 27 (1986): 621.

17. Candace B. Pert et al., "Neuropeptides and Their Receptors: A Psychosomatic Network," *Journal of Immunology* 135 (suppl.), (1985): 820.

18. Esther M. Sternberg, *Healing Spaces* (Belknap Press of Harvard University Press: Cambridge, 2009).

19. Siegel, *Love, Medicine, and Miracles.*

20. Pedro Lain Entralgo, *The Therapy of the Word in Classical Antiquity* (Yale University Press: New Haven, 1970).

21. H. M. Spiro, "Placebos, Patients, and Physicians" in *In Search of the Modern Hippocrates* (University of Iowa Press: Iowa City, 1987).

22. A. Kirkley et al., "A Randomized Trial of Arthroscopic Surgery for Osteoarthritis of the Knee," *New England Journal of Medicine*, 359, no. 11 (2008): 1097–1107.

23. Harris Gardiner, "Study Finds Many Doctors Give Placebos," *New York Times*, Oct. 24, 2008, A-12.

24. W. M. Zinn, "Transference Phenomena in Medical Practice: Being Whom the Patient Needs," *Annals of Internal Medicine* 113 (1990): 293.

25. Spiro, "Placebos, Patients, and Physicians."

Chapter 4. Understanding Suffering

1. E. J. Cassell, "The Nature of Suffering: Physical, Psychological, Social, and Spiritual Aspects," in *The Hidden Dimension of Illness: Human Suffering*, (National Leagues of Nursing Press: New York, 1992).

2. M. Osterweis, F. Solomon, and M. Green, eds. *Bereavement: Reactions, Consequences, and Care* (National Academy Press: Washington, DC, 1984).

3. Herman Feifel, ed. *The Meaning of Death* (McGraw-Hill: New York, 1959).

4. John E. Fortunato, *AIDS: The Spiritual Dilemma* (Harper & Row: New York, 1987).

5. Richard F. Vieth, *Holy Power: Human Pain* (Meyer Stone: Bloomington, IN, 1988).

6. Margaret Mead, *Culture and Commitment* (Doubleday: New York, 1970).

7. Howard Brody, *Stories of Sickness* (Yale University Press: New Haven, 1987).

8. Drew Gilpin Faust, *The Republic of Suffering* (Knopf: New York, 2008).

9. Arthur Kleinman, *The Illness Narratives: Suffering, Healing and the Human Condition* (Basic Books: New York, 1988), 23.

10. Bellah et. al., *Habits of the Heart*.

11. Cassell, "The Nature of Suffering."

12. E. Heitman, "The Influence of Values and Culture in Response to Suffering," *The Hidden Dimension of Illness: Human Suffering* (National League for Nursing Press: New York, 1992).

13. Donald Seldin, "The Boundaries of Medicine," *Transactions of the Association of American Physicians* 97 (1981): 75–84.

14. Kleinman, *The Illness Narratives*.

15. William F. May, *The Patient's Ordeal* (Indiana University Press: Bloomington, IN, 1991).

16. Patricia L. Starck and John P. McGovern, eds. *The Hidden Dimension of Illness: Human Suffering* (National League for Nursing Press: New York, 1992).

17. Robert Augros, *The New Biology: Discovering the Wisdom of Nature* (New Science Library: Boston, 1987).

18. Margaret Gerteis et al., eds., *Through the Patient's Eyes: Understanding and Promoting Patient-Centered Care* (Josey-Bass Publishers: San Francisco, 1993).

19. J. Santo, "Let the Patients Decide," *Consumer Reports*, December 2008, 13.

20. Brody, *Stories of Sickness*.

Chapter 5. Where Life and Death Meet

1. R. J. Bulger, "The Dying Patient and His Doctor," *Harvard Medical Bulletin*, April 1960, 23–25, 45–47.

2. Outlook, *New York Times*, Jan. 11, 2009, B1, B4.

3. Ibid.

4. Sherwin B. Nuland, *How We Die: Reflections on Life's Final Chapter* (Knopf: New York, 1993).

5. Siegel, *Love, Medicine, and Miracles*.

6. Nuland, *How We Die*.

7. Timothy E. Quill, *Death and Dignity: Making Choices and Taking Charge* (W.W. Norton & Company: New York, 1992).

8. Nuland, *How We Die*.

9. Bulger, "The Dying Patient and His Doctor."

10. Daniel Callahan, *The Troubled Dream of Life: Living with Mortality* (Simon & Schuster: New York, 1993).

11. Ibid.

12. Quill, *Death and Dignity.*

13. Elizabeth Kübler-Ross, *On Death and Dying* (Macmillan: New York, 1969).

14. Timothy E. Quill, "Doctor, I Want to Die," *Journal of the American Medical Association* 270 (1993): 870–873.

15. Nuland, *How We Die.*

16. Quill, "Doctor I Want to Die."

17. Ibid.

18. E. Pellegrino, "Compassion Needs Reason Too," *Journal of the American Medical Association* 270 (1993): 874–875.

19. Pauline Chen, *Final Exam: A Surgeon's Reflections on Mortality* (Vintage Books: New York, 2008).

20. Quill, "Doctor I Want to Die."

21. Pellegrino, "Compassion Needs Reason Too."

22. John J. McDermott, *Streams of Experience* (University of Massachusetts Press, Amherst, 1986).

23. Ibid.

24. See www.ErnestBeckerFoundation.org; Ernst Becker, *The Denial of Death* (Simon & Shuster: New York, 1973).

25. Richard Dawkins, *The God Delusion* (Houghton Mifflin Books: New York, 2006).

26. Ernst Becker, *Escape from Evil* (Free Press: New York, 1975).

27. John Updike, "Requiem," op-ed, *New York Times*, January 28, 2009.

28. Alan Brown. Announcement of his death to author, 2007.

Chapter 6. Unity and Divsersity with Patients and Populations

1. E. D. Mintz and R. Guerrant, "Global Health: A Lion in Our Village: The Unconscionable Tragedy of Cholera in Africa," *New England Journal of Medicine* 360, no. 11, 2009, 1060–1062.

2. Institute of Medicine, *The Future of Public Health* (National Academy Press: Washington DC, 1988).

3. Ibid.

4. Koch's postulates continue to underlie the study of infectious diseases. Koch postulated that the same pathogen must be present in every case of the disease, must be isolated from the diseased host, and a pure culture of the pathogen must cause the disease upon inoculation into a susceptible laboratory animal.

5. Institute of Medicine, *The Future of Public Health*.

6. Elizabeth Fee, *Disease and Discovery: A History of the Johns Hopkins School of Hygiene and Public Health, 1916–1939* (Johns Hopkins University Press: Baltimore, 1987).

7. Kerr L. White and Julia E. Connelly, eds., *The Medical School's Mission and the Population's Health* (Springer-Verlag: New York, 1992).

8. Institute of Medicine, *The Future of Public Health*.

9. Paul Starr, *The Social Transformation of American Medicine* (Basic Books: New York, 1982), 187.

10. R. J. Bulger, "Reductionist Biology and Population Medicine: Strange Bedfellows or a Marriage Made in Heaven?," editorial, *Journal of the American Medical Association* 264, 508–509.

11. R. S. Lawrence, "The Role of Physicians in Promoting Health," *Health Affairs* (Summer 1990), 122–132.

12. Ibid.

13. White and Connelly, eds. *The Medical School's Mission*.

14. Ibid.

15. Lawrence, "The Role of Physicians in Promoting Health."

16. R. J. Pels, D. H. Bor, and R. S. Lawrence, "Decision Making for Introducing Preventive Clinical Services," *Annual Review of Public Health* 10 (1989): 359–379.

17. L. Eisenberg, "Science in Medicine: Too Much to Too Little and Too Limited in Scope?" in *The Task of Medicine: Dialogue at Wickenburg* (Henry J. Kaiser Family Foundation: Menlo Park, 1988).

18. White and Connelly, eds. *The Medical School's Mission*.

19. J. K. Iglehart, "Perspectives of an Errant Economist: A Conversation with Tom Schelling," *Health Affairs* (Summer 1990), 109–122.

20. Lawrence, "The Role of Physicians in Promoting Health."

21. R. C. Henry, K. S. Ogle, and L. A. Snellman, "Preventive Medicine: Physician Practices, Beliefs, and Perceived Barriers for Implementation," *Family Medicine* 19 (1987): 100–113.

22. H. Wechsler, S. Levine, R. K. Idelson, M. Rohman, and J. O. Taylor, "The

Physician's Role in Health Promotion: A Survey of Primary Care Practitioners," *New England Journal of Medicine* 308 (1996): 97–100.

23. M. B. Johns, M. F. Hovell, T. Ganiats, K. M. Peddecord, and W. S. Agras, "Primary Care and Health Promotion: A Model for Preventive Medicine," *American Journal of Preventive Medicine* 6 (1987): 346–358.

24. D. H. Gemson and J. Elinson, "Prevention in Primary Care: Variability in Physician Practice Patterns in New York City," *American Journal of Preventive Medicine* 2 (1986): 226–234.

25. Lawrence, "The Role of Physicians in Promoting Health."

26. Ibid.

27. J. R. Evans, "The 'Health of the Public' Approach to Medical Education," *Academic Medicine* 67 (1992): 719–723.

28. Bulger, "Reductionist Biology and Population Medicine."

29. L. Breslow, "A Health Promotion Primer for the 1990s," *Health Affairs* (Summer 1990): 6–21.

30. Institute of Medicine, *Unequal Treatment: Confronting Racial and Ethnic Disparities in Health Care* (National Academy Press: Washington, DC, 2003).

31. David Satcher and Rubens Pamies, *Multicultural Medicine and Health Disparities* (McGraw Hill: New York, 2006).

32. Richard A. Williams, *Eliminating Health Care Disparities in America* (Humana Press: Totowa, NJ, 2007).

33. Iglehart, "Perspectives of an Errant Economist."

34. Institute of Medicine Roundtable on Environmental Health Sciences, Research and Medicine; meeting held April 8, 2008, Paul Rogers and Lynn Goldman, co-chairs.

35. A. D. Tsouros et al., eds. "Health Promoting Universities: Concept, Experience, and Framework for Action," World Health Organization, 1998.

Chapter 7. On Serving and Collaborating

1. Guido Majno, "The Lost Secret of Ancient Medicine," *In Search of the Modern Hippocrates* (University of Iowa Press: Iowa City, 1987).

2. Ibid.

3. Gabriel Marcel, *Man against Mass Society* (Henry Regency Co.; Chicago, 1962).

4. Robert Coles, *The Call of Service: A Witness to Idealism* (Houghton-Mifflin: Boston, 1993).

5. Ibid.

6. Nuland, *How We Die.*

7. Tracy Thompson, *The Beast: A Journey Through Depression* (Penguin: London, 1996).

8. D. Beatrice, C. Thomas, B. Biles, "Grant-Making with an Impact: The Picker-Commonwealth Patient-Centered Care Program," *Health Affairs* 17 no. 1 (Jan.–Feb. 1998), 236–244.

9. John J. Nance, *Why Hospitals Should Fly: The Ultimate Flight Plan to Patient Safety and Quality Care* (Second River Health Care Press: Bozeman, MT, 2008).

10. David Lawrence, *From Chaos to Care: The Promise of Team-Based Medicine* (Perseus: Cambridge, 2002).

Chapter 8. Three Paradigms for Education and Practice

1. George L. Engel, "How Much Longer Must Medicine's Science Be Bound by a Seventeenth Century World View?" in *The Task of Medicine* (Henry J. Kaiser Foundation: Menlo Park, 1988).

2. Havens, *Making Contact.*

3. L. Eisenberg, "Science in Medicine: Too Much to Too Little and Too Limited in Scope?," *The Task of Medicine: Dialogue at Wickenburg*(Henry J. Kaiser Family Foundation: Menlo Park, 1988).

4. Kleinman, *The Illness Narratives.*

Chapter 9. Covenants, Commitment, and Tragic Choices

1. E. D. Pellegrino, "Toward an Expanded Medical Ethics: The Hippocratic Oath Revisited" in *Hippocrates Revisited* (University of Iowa Press: Iowa City, 1987).

2. Ibid.

3. William F. May, *The Physician's Covenant: Images of the Healer in Medical Ethics* (Westminster Press: Philadelphia, 1983).

4. R. J. Bulger, "Dialogue with Hippocrates and Griff T. Ross" in *Search for the Modern Hippocrates* (University of Iowa Press: Iowa City, 1988).

5. Edmund D. Pellegrino and David C. Thomasma, *For the Patient's Good: The Restoration of Beneficence in Health Care* (Oxford University Press: New York, 1988).

6. J. Darley and C. D. Batson, "From Jerusalem to Jericho: A Study of Situational and Dispositional Variables in Helping Behavior," *Journal of Personality and Social Psychology* 27 (1973): 100–108.

7. Kenneth Ludmerer, *Learning to Heal: The Development of American Medical Education* (Basic Books: New York, 1985).

8. Kenneth Ludmerer, *Time to Heal: American Medical Education from the Turn of the Century to the Era of Managed Care* (Oxford University Press: New York, 1999).

9. BBC News, "A Mother's Race against Time," http://news.bbc.co.uk /2/hi/africa/8320781.stm.

Chapter 10. Measuring American Health Care with Human Values

1. U.S. Congress's "Mr. Health" (1921–2008; member of the U.S. House of Representatives from Florida, 1955–1979).

2. Cochrane is an internationally known health analyst; from a speech given in 1972 Washington, DC.

3. R. J. Bulger, "On Hippocrates, Thomas Jefferson and Max Weber: The Bureaucratic, Technological Imperatives and the Future of the Healing Tradition in the Voluntary Society" in *The Tanner Lectures on Human Values* (University of Utah Press: Salt Lake City, 1980).

4. Jay Katz, *The Silent World of the Doctor and Patient* (Free Press: New York, 1984).

5. A. S. Relman, "The New Medical-Industrial Complex," *New England Journal of Medicine* 303 no. 17, (1980): 963–970.

6. Jerome P. Kassirer, *On The Take: How Medicine's Complicity with Big Business Can Endanger Your Health* (Oxford University Press: London, 2005).

7. Peter Gosselin, *High Wire: The Precarious Financial Lives of American Families* (Basic Books: New York, 2007).

8. William May, *The Physician's Covenant* (Westminster Press: Philadelphia, 2000).

9. Eric J. Cassell, *The Nature of Suffering and the Goals of Medicine*, Oxford University Press: New York, 1991).

10. Patricia L. Starck and John P. McGovern, eds. *The Hidden Dimension of Illness: Human Suffering* (National League for Nursing Press: New York, 1992).

11. Ruth Bulger and Stanley A. Reiser, *Integrity in Health Care Institutions: Humane Environments for Teaching, Inquiry, and Healing* (University of Iowa Press: Iowa City, 1990).

12. Personal communication from Michael Maccoby, 2001.

13. R. J. Bulger, "What Will Health Care Look Like in the Future?" in *Creating Nursing's Future* (Mosby: St. Louis, 1999), 14–31.

14. McDermott, *Streams of Experience.*

15. R. J. Bulger, *Technology, Bureaucracy and Healing in America: A Postmodern Paradigm* (University of Iowa Press: Iowa City, 1988).

16. K. Brewster, "The Voluntary Society" in *The Tanner Lectures on Human Values VIII* (University of Utah Press: Salt Lake City, 1983), 1–41.

17. Ralf Dahrendorf, *Life Chances: Approaches to Social and Political Theory,* (Weidenfeld & Nicholson: London, 1979).

18. Thomas P. McDonnell, *Thomas Merton Reader* (Image Books: Garden City, 1974).

19. Oscar Handlin, *The Uprooted,* second ed. (Atlantic-Little Brown, Boston, 1973).

20. Bellah et al., *Habits of the Heart.*

21. Daniel J. Boorstin, *Hidden History.*

22. Margaret Gerteis et al., eds. *Through the Patient's Eyes.*

23. C. S. Bosk, "The Transformation of the Therapeutic Relationship" in *The Digital Decade: Promise and Peril for the Academic Health Center,* Association of Academic Health Centers: Washington, DC, 1997).

24. Cohen, *Strong at the Broken Places.*

25. Jim Collins, *Good to Great* (HarperBussiness: New York, 2001).

Acknowledgments

Beginning with my first published paper, "Doctors and Dying," written in 1958, and continuing throughout my more than half-century involvement with medicine and health care, I have tried to keep focused on the human goals and values intrinsic to the healing and caring enterprise, even in this most technological of times. I have worked with and learned from many colleagues, friends, and teachers throughout the years, including my wife, Ruth, a prominent scientist and teacher-ethicist.

However, it must be said that the work that went into this book had its roots in two developments: the formation, in the mid-1960s, of the Society for Health and Human Values; and the 1972 addition of a section on health and human values as a core of the earliest program plan established to guide the efforts of the new Institute of Medicine of the National Academy of Sciences. As a young academic physician I was privileged to participate in the early stages of both organizations. Subsequently, I tried to bring the perspectives and lessons I learned to academic jobs in various parts of the country

Thus, I owe whatever is instructive, relevant, or interesting in the following pages to too many people to identify here. It is well to express my gratitude to three groups of people. The first of these groups must be the two foundations that invested in my work in these areas over the last thirty years. The first is the John McGovern Foundation, which has faithfully given substantial fiscal and moral support to the human values issues within range of the institutions at which I worked, beginning in 1978 at the University of Texas Health Science Center at Houston. Even after I retired from the Association of Academic Health Centers (AAHC) in 2005 and after Dr. McGovern's death, the foundation he started and developed provided much-needed support for the writing and preparing of this manuscript for publication. The Josiah Macy Foundation, also a long-standing supporter of the policy and substantive issues surrounding the education of health professionals and of the AAHC, at which I worked for seventeen years, also made a generous grant to add to that of the McGovern Foundation, making possible the final evolution and shaping of the manuscript.

My appreciation is also extended to my colleagues on the Board of Directors of the AAHC for encouraging the pursuit of our exploration of the concept of the Organizational Therapeutic Index, which I have modified further recently in the appendix of this book, as an example of how it is possible to measure success in living up to professional and organizational ideals and values.

The second group needing mention and requiring gratitude includes the many mentors, teachers, colleagues, and exemplars whose work and professional example helped me to keep learning. They are exemplified in the names listed in the dedication. I thank them all! The third important group consists of those who helped significantly in the production of the final manuscript. Marian Osterweis, PhD, a gifted and knowledgeable sociologist and writer, offered many useful suggestions and criticism early on. Faith and Grace, my two daughters, each played a role in contributing ideas and words. Grace actually resurrected the project by bringing forth an otherwise forgotten original text from some years previously that Elizabeth Bobby (then a research assistant in my office) and I had developed. The subject of this text dealt with aspects of what is now chapter 2, "Healing with Technology and with Words, Art, and the Senses". I could not have managed the computer dimensions of preparing the manuscript for my editor, Hilary Hinzmann, if my wife hadn't essentially taken it over from me after I repeatedly sent whole paragraphs of my timeless prose into infinity, never to return. The truth is that Hilary finally got hold of the manuscript and cajoled, required, added, subtracted, and smoothed the text into what now seems a coherent set of ideas. Perhaps they were all there somewhere, but what he taught me was that in order to attract a reader I needed to scour my memory for personal stories to illustrate the issue or subject I was about to introduce. His scope of learning and intelligence were manifest to me, but his insistence on personal stories has brought new life to the talks I still give, as well as to the manuscript. In sum, I greatly appreciate what he has done. I was fortunate to find someone adept not only with the world of science but also with the world of human interaction, including the handling of disease and the suffering it entails. Gray Cutler helped greatly with her assiduous copyediting. David Wilk, a publishing guru, in addition to persuading Hilary Hinzmann to take me under his wing, guided the whole process of bringing the manuscript to publication. And finally, I never would have found David and Hilary if my friend Yousaif August had not arranged for Eugene Schwartz to read the manuscript and to agree to point me somewhere. The only credit I might deserve is for being smart enough to do exactly what Eugene told me to do.

About the Author

Dr. Roger J. Bulger, an academic physician, researcher, educator, administrator, and lately a patient, has spent his career exploring the connections among human values, health care and health policy. Dr. Bulger served three times as the chairman of Institute of Medicine Study Committees, each of which in turn produced major book-length policy studies published by the National Academies Press. Their titles were: *Medical Professional Liability and the Delivery of Obstetrical Care* (1989), *Health Data in the Information Age: Use, Disclosure and Privacy* (1994), *Leading Health Indicators for Healthy People 2010* (1999).